Obesity Research

Obesity Research

Published by iConcept Press

Obesity Research

Publisher: iConcept Press Ltd.

ISBN: 978-1-922227-67-6

Printed in the United States of America

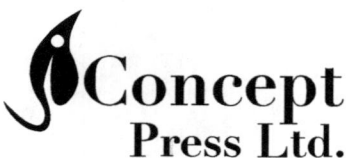

ıꞋConcept
Press Ltd.

www.iconceptpress.com

Contents

Preface

Obesity is a major contributor to serious health conditions including type-2 diabetes, cardiovascular disease and arthritis. It is a major threat to the health across all ages, races, and socioeconomic groups, and in particular within disadvantaged and underserved communities. Promoting healthy weight requires concerted efforts, including quality improvement, from health care, public health and communities. This book offers prompt publication of original research and presents new information. Specifically, the intent is to address the following areas with respect to obesity prevention: potential interventions, bariatric surgery, arthritis, type 1 and 2 diabetes mellitus, hypercholesterolemia and atherosclerosis.

In Chapter 1, the authors review comparative prevalence of obesity and its trend in Canada, various determinants and risk factors, and potential strategies for its prevention. Chapter 2 synthesizes school-based obesity prevention interventions which incorporate environmental change. Recommendations for the development of future multi-component interventions which incorporate environmental change are provided. Chapter 3 reviews the latest literature on the cost effectiveness of bariatric surgery. Analysis shows that bariatric surgery is cost effective compared to conventional treatment or no treatment, particularly in severely obese and diabetic patients with convincing incremental cost-utility ratios (ICUR) ranging from $1,000–$40,000 per quality adjusted life years. Chapter 4 discusses the use of biologics for management of Rheumatoid Arthritis (RA). RA is a chronic, frequently progressive, and destructive autoimmune disease. As the disease progresses, irreversible joint damage may lead to loss of function and physical disability. Since this disease cannot be cured, management of this disease becomes an important endeavor with the aim of inducing and maintaining remission, and altering the course of disease.

Chapter 5 with the prevention of spinal glial activation by fluorocitrate in an attempt to maintain prolonged pain relief and the prevention of opioid dependence. It discusses the possibility that the analgesic effect of fluorocitrate intratecal (i.t.) administration in a rat model of experimental arthritis can be possibly modulated by the i.t. administration of D-serine. Chapter 6 proposes that "Lean type 2 diabetes" is a distinct and fairly common clinical entity reported across the globe. It discusses the difference in pathophysiology and complication of lean type 2 diabetes from the obese. Chapter 7 proposes that Dermcidin isoform-2, a stress protein induced acute coronary syntrome through the mediation of diabetes, hypertension and hyperchlosterolemia which are the leading cause of atherosclerosis in the disease.

Editing and publishing a book is never an easy task. Each chapter in this book has gone through a peer review, a selection and an editing process so as to guarantee its quality. Without the supports and contributions of the authors and reviewers, this book can never be able to complete. We would like to thank all of the authors in this book and all of the reviewers who participated in the reviewing process: Rieke Alten, Katarína Bauerová, Barbara M. Brooks-Worrell, Marcelo Diarcadia Mariano Cezar, Chih-Cheng Chen, Hongping Chen, Palma Chillón, Min Chul Cho, Anne Dee, Wilhelmina C. M. Duivenvoorden, Emmanouil Giorgakis, Jeffrey W. Grimm, Aldric Hama, Kenji Hashimoto, Jer-Yiing Houng, Anup Katheria, Parjeet Kaur, Nam Kyu Kim, Mikhail M Kostik, Jian-Fang Li, Ying-Ming Liou, Tomoko Matsumoto, Camila Moreno Rosa Bassetto, Gisela Nyberg, Marina P. Okoshi, Tong Peijian, Raghavendra Pralhada Rao, Shelly Russell-Mayhew, Toshio Tanaka, Wendy Van Lippevelde, Cecilia Vecoli, Eva M Vivian, Daorong Wang and Hana Yoon. We hope that you, the reader, will find this book interesting and useful. Any advices please feel free and are always welcome to tell us.

iConcept Press Editorial Office
July 2016

Chapter 1

Obesity in Canada: Prevalence, Determinants and Potential Interventions

Rabia K. Shahid[1], Shahid Ahmed[1]

1 Introduction

Obesity has become a global public health problem. Over the past decades its prevalence has increased in different populations. It has been associated with significant morbidity and mortality (Pi-Sunyer, 1993; Visscher & Visscher, 2001). It is well recognized that obesity increases the risk of various chronic illnesses such as type II diabetes, cardiovascular disease, hypertension, cerebro-vascular accident, gallbladder disease, osteoarthritis, sleep apnea and several cancers (Field *et al.*, 2001; Lukanova *et al.*, 2006; Must *et al.*, 1999; Pi-Sunyer, 1993; Visscher & Visscher, 2001). It also affects the mental health. Health care costs are considerably higher for overweight and obese individuals (Pi-Sunyer, 1993; Visscher & Visscher, 2001). The increasing burden of obesity and its associated comorbid illnesses result in an increasing threat to both the overall health status of Canadians and the Canadian healthcare system. In this paper we review risk factors and determinants of obesity, its prevalence in Canada, and potential interventions to prevent it.

1.1 Definitions

The National Heart, Lung, and Blood Institute and the World Health Organization (WHO) have provided uniform definitions of overweight and obesity (National Institutes of Health. National Heart, Lung, and Blood Institute, 1998; WHO, 1998). Although "overweight" technically refers to an excess of body weight and "obesity" to an excess

---

[1] Medicine and Epidemiology and Community Health, University of Saskatchewan, Saskatoon, SK, Canada

of fat, these two words can be defined operationally in terms of the body mass index (BMI). The degree of risk associated with overweight is related to the BMI. A BMI between 25 and 30 kg/m^2 is low risk, above 30 kg/m^2 is moderate risk. The WHO and the National Center for Health Statistics define overweight as a BMI > 25 and ≤ 29.9 and obesity as a BMI greater than 30 kg/m^2.

2   Etiology and Natural History of Obesity

Several factors contribute to the development of obesity. Among them, lifestyle and diet are the most important risk factors. People can get obese at any age; however, there are certain times when they are more prone to gain weight.

2.1   Prenatal Influences

High caloric intake by mother, maternal smoking and diabetes during pregnancy increase the risk of heavy offspring and obesity later in life (Power & Jefferis, 2002).

2.2   Breastfeeding

Breastfeeding when compared to formula milk is associated with lower risk of overweight. Several studies have shown that feeding infants solely with breast milk during first three or more months of life reduces the risk of being overweight later in the childhood (Gillman *et al.*, 2001; Hediger *et al.*, 2001).

2.3   Childhood & Adolescence

The predictive value of childhood obesity varies with age of onset of obesity and family history. It has been reported that obese children under three years of age are at low risk of becoming obese adults unless one or both parents are obese. On the other hand, obesity among older children is an increasingly important predictor of adult obesity (The *et al.*, 2010; Whitaker *et al.*, 1997). Likewise, obesity in adolescence is associated with severe obesity in adult.

2.4   Adult Women & Men

The long-term risk of getting obese or overweight in the adulthood seems to be very high. In a prospective cohort study, 14 to 19 percent of women and 26 to 30 percent of men who were normal weight at baseline became overweight within four years of enrollment into the study (Aloia *et al.*, 1995). Most overweight women gain weight after puberty. The weight gain may be precipitated by number of factors, including pregnancy, oral contraceptive and menopause (Aloia *et al.*, 1995; Bray & Bellanger, 2006). In men, transition from active lifestyle during the teens and twenties to a more sedentary lifestyle thereafter is associated with weight gain (Bray & Bellanger, 2006).

2.5   Life Style and Diet

A low level of physical activity is strongly correlated with weight gain and obesity in both men and women. Sedentary lifestyle lowers energy expenditure thereby promotes weight gain. Epidemiological data support that various dietary habits including a diet high in fat, overeating, night-eating syndrome and frequent fast-food consumption are associated with obesity (Bray & Bellanger, 2006; Christakis & Fowler, 2007; Flegal *et al.*, 1995; Lawson *et al.*, 1995; Mozaffarian *et al.*, 2011; Vasan *et al.*, 2005). Furthermore, evidence suggests that sleeps deprivation could result in excessive eating, obesity, and altered response to dietary therapy (Christakis & Fowler, 2007).

2.6   Drug Induced Obesity

A number of drugs such as antipsychotics, antidepressants, antiepileptic drugs, antihyperglycemic agents, and hormones can cause weight gain and obesity (Leslie *et al.*, 2007).

2.7   Neuroendocrine Obesity

Several neuroendocrine disorders including Cushing's syndrome, hypothyroidism, polycystic ovary syndrome, and excess growth hormone are associated with the development of obesity (Hochberg & Hochberg, 2010).

3   Prevalence in Canada

Obesity is expected to surpass smoking as the leading cause of preventable morbidity and mortality. The prevalence of obesity has been rising in Canada. According to measured height and weight data from 2007–2009 about one in four Canadian adults are obese, nearly 10% higher than in 1978 when obesity rate was 13.8% (Shields *et al.*, 2010; Statistics Canada, 2009; 2010; The Public Health Agency of Canada, 2011) (Figure 1). When obesity was combined with overweight, self-reported prevalence of obesity and overweight was 51.1% compared with 62.1% when measured data was used. Of children and youth aged six to seventeen, 8.6% are obese.

Self reported obesity rates are usually underreported. According to measured height and weight data from 2007–2009, 17.4% people reported to be obese (Statistics Canada, 2010). Self-reported obesity across the health regions within Canada is 5.3% to 35.9%. It is more prevalent among Aboriginals peoples than in the non-Aboriginal adult population. For example, 25.7% off-reserve Aboriginal adults reported to be obese compared with 17.4% non-Aboriginal adults in Canada (The Public Health Agency of Canada, 2011). First Nations on reserve have higher prevalence of 36%. The prevalence in men and women is almost similar and is approximately 22%. The prevalence increases with age, peaking in people who are 55 to 64 years old (Figure 2). Of note, obesity rate declines sharply after the age of 75 (The Public Health Agency of Canada, 2011)

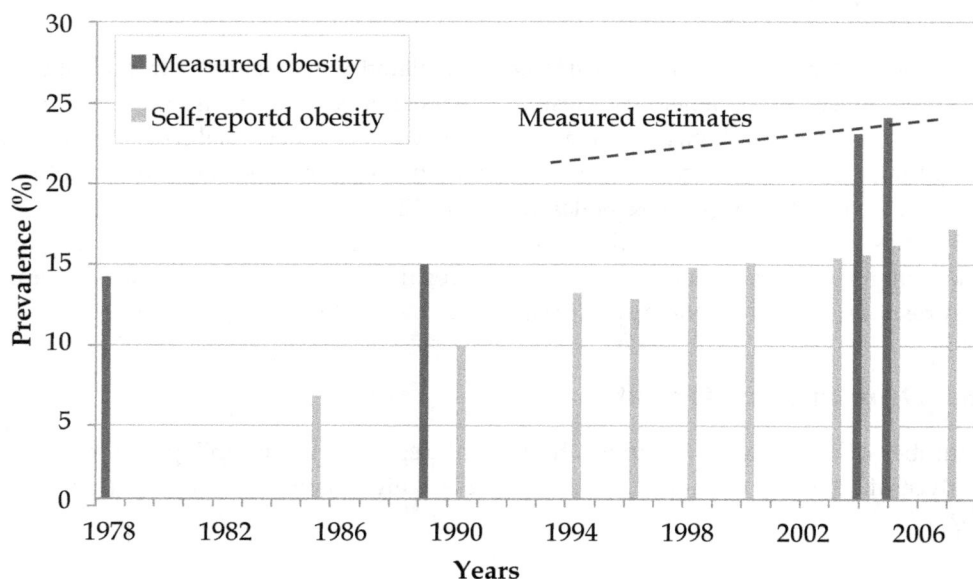

Figure 1: Percentage of the population age eighteen years or above, who were obese (measured and self-reported), by year, in Canada during the period of 1978–2007. Source Public Health Agency of Canada. http://www.phac-aspc.gc.ca

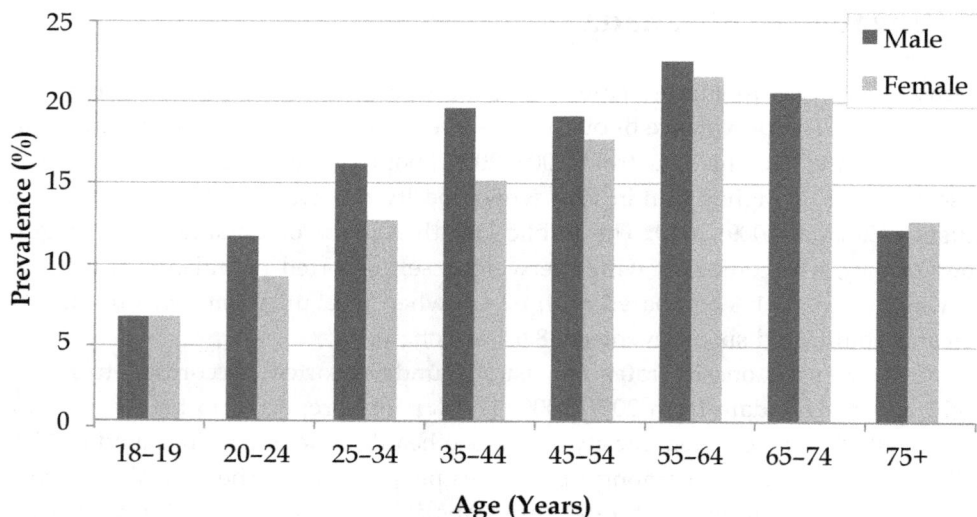

Figure 2: Prevalence of self-reported obesity among men and women eighteen years and older, by age group, 2007. Source Public Health Agency of Canada. http://www.phac-aspc.gc.ca

The 2007–2009 Canadian Health Measure Survey (CHMS) revealed that an average 45-year old man was about 9.2 kg (20 pounds) heavier than his 1981 counterpart. Since height was not significantly different, the BMI increased by more than 2 kg/m². The waist circumference of an average 45-year old man has increased by 6.4 cm (2.5 inches) (Statistics Canada, 2010).

An average 45-year old woman weight has increased by 5.2 kg (12 pounds), while height has stayed relatively constant over the period. As a result, the BMI has increased by 2 kg/m², shifting her from normal weight to the overweight category. The waist circumference has increased by 7.1 cm (2.8 inches) (Statistics Canada, 2010). Independent of age and sex, a large percentage of adults had suboptimal health benefit ratings for all the fitness components. According to 2007–2009 CHMS average man "grip strength" rating decreased from very good to good, while his "sit-and-reach" score was slightly higher compared with 1981 survey. Though average woman grip strength decreased, her flexibility was approximately the same in 2007–2009 CHMS (Statistics Canada, 2010).

3.1   Variation by age and sex

According to 2004 and 2007–2008 Canadian Community Health Survey (CCHS), the prevalence of obesity increases in both men and women up to age 65 and declines in people older than 65. Based on self-reported data, the obesity was more prevalent among men than women (Figure 2). Based on direct measures, in population aged 20 to 39, 19% of males and 21% of females were obese and among aged 40 to 59, 27% of males and 24% of females were obese (Shields *et al.*, 2010; Statistics Canada, 2010; The Public Health Agency of Canada, 2011). It was not consistently higher among men than women.

3.2   Provincial and Territorial Variation

The rates of obesity are different across various provinces and territories (Figure 3). As per 2007–2008 CCHS, the prevalence of self-reported obesity was 12.8% in British Columbia and approximately 25% in Newfoundland and Labrador. Estimates of obesity in 2007–2008 survey were found to be significantly higher overall in Canada as well as in Alberta and Ontario than 2005 survey and significantly higher in 2005 than 2003 in Newfoundland and Labrador.

3.3   Prevalence among aboriginal

First Nations people who lived off- reserve and Métis people were more likely than the non-Aboriginal population to be physically active in their leisure time: 37% and 39% versus 30%. However, the percentage of Inuit who were physically active (31%) was not significantly different from the percentage for non-Aboriginal people (Shields *et al.*, 2010; Statistics Canada, 2009; 2010). Despite that self-reported obesity is more prevalent among Aboriginal people (Elgar & Stewart, 2008; First Nations Centre, 2005).

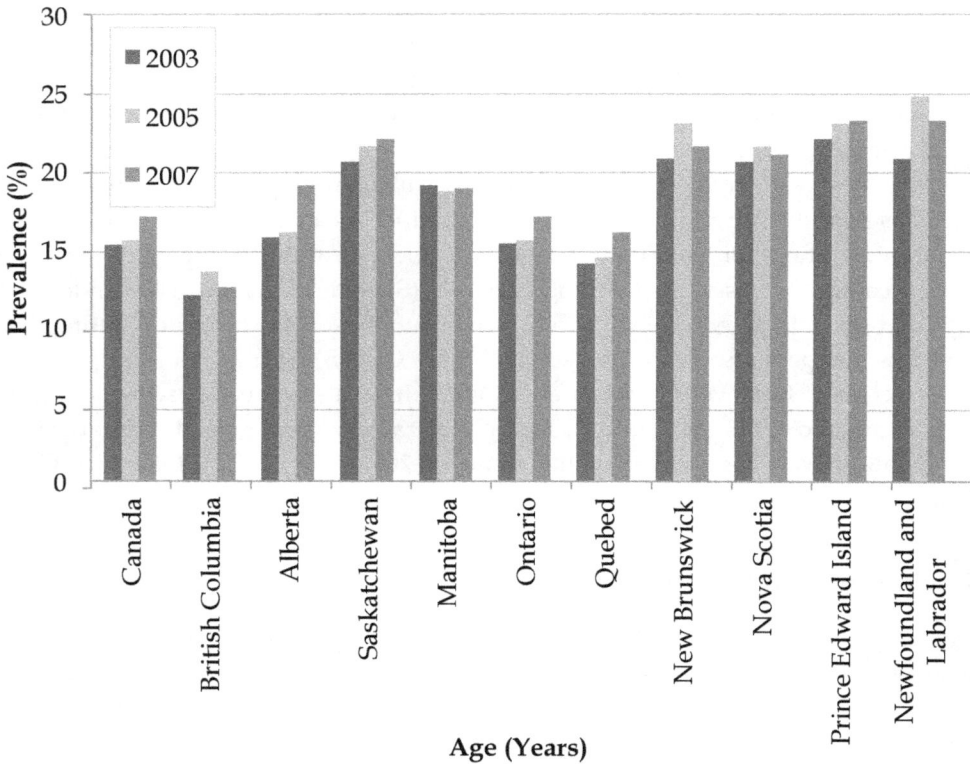

Figure 3: Prevalence of Self-Reported Obesity among People 18 Years and Older, by Province, and Year. Source Public Health Agency of Canada. http://www. phac-aspc.gc.ca

3.4 First Nations off-reserve:

According to 2007/08 CCHS, 25.7% of Aboriginal adults (excluding First Nations on-reserve) were obese. This is comparable to the results of 2006 Aboriginal Peoples Survey (APS), which revealed a self reported prevalence of 26.1%. Similar to general population, prevalence of obesity among Aboriginal with self-reported data is lower than measured data (Statistics Canada, 2009). For example, according to 2004 CCHS 37.8% of off-reserve Aboriginal adults were obese on the basis of measured heights and weights, compared with 25.7% as per self-reported data.

3.5 First Nations On-reserve:

Analysis of the First Nations Regional Longitudinal Health Survey (RHS) showed the prevalence of obesity is 36.0% among adults on reserve (31.8% of males and 41.4% of females) (Elgar & Stewart, 2008; First Nations Centre, 2005).

According to the 2006 APS, prevalence of obesity in the Métis population was 26.4% among adults whereas 23.9% Inuit adults were reported to be obese (Statistics Canada, 2009).

3.6   Regional Variation

Studies have found that the prevalence of obesity tends to be lower in more urban regions. For example, the 2003 CCHS revealed that obesity was significantly below the national average in Montreal, Toronto and Vancouver. In both adults and youth, the proportion of being overweight inclines to be higher in rural areas than in metropolitan areas (Statistics Canada, 2010; The Public Health Agency of Canada, 2011).

4   Changes in the Prevalence Over Time

4.1   Worldwide

In recent decades, obesity has turned into a major global issue. The WHO has estimated that more than 1 billion adults worldwide are overweight and at least 300 million are clinically obese (WHO, 1998).

The measured obesity varies from 3.4% in Japan to 34.3% in the United Stated. Obesity has increased among men and women between 1980s and 2005 in countries like Canada, Australia, England, France, Hungary and United States. Researchers are also anticipating increase in Canada, Australia, England and United States until 2019.

4.2   Changes over time in Canada

Both measured and self-reported data have shown an increased in the prevalence of obesity in adults aged 18 or older. Obesity rates are high in Canada compared to Organization for Economic Cooperation & Development (OECD) countries but they have not increased substantially in the last 15 years (Figure 4). Two out of 3 men are overweight and 1 in 4 people are obese in Canada, but overall the rate of increase has been one of the slowest in the OECD countries. The OECD has projected that proportion of overweight people will rise 5% during the next 10 years.

4.3   Changes over time in Aboriginal people

Limited data are available to examine changes in obesity prevalence over time in Aboriginal populations (Nolin *et al.*, 2004). On the basis of measured data, it has been estimated that obesity prevalence among adult's ages 18–74 has increased by 49% (from 19% to 28%). Although prevalence has increased in both sexes, the increase was more significant among males than females (73% increase vs. 31% increase, respectively) (Statistics Canada, 2010; The Public Health Agency of Canada, 2011).

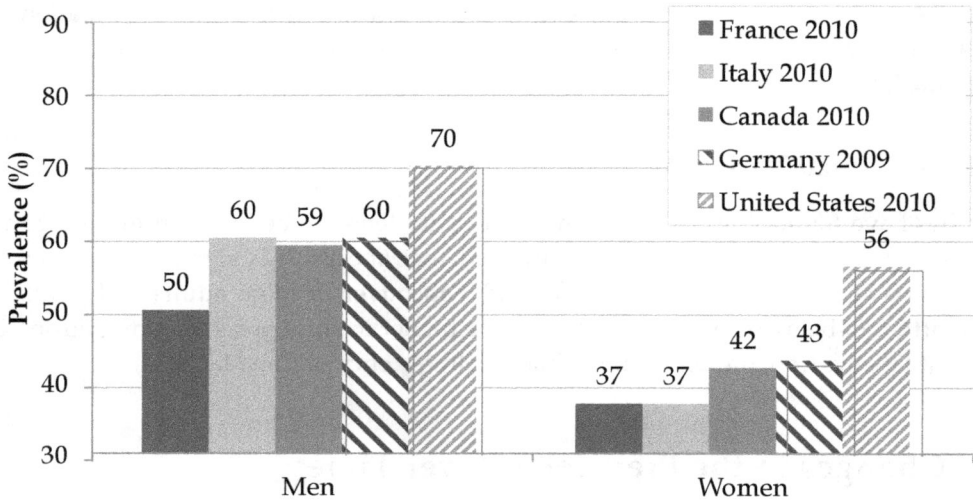

Figure 4: Rates of overweight and obesity in G-7 countries in 2009–2010. Source: Organization for Economic Co-operation and Development (OECD). OECD Health data 2012. OECD Statistics.

5   Differences in Obesity Prevalence Estimates between Canada and the United States

In 2007–2009, the prevalence of obesity in Canada was 25.6 %; over 7 percentage points lower than the prevalence of 33 % in the United States (Figure 5). Among men, the prevalence of obesity was over 5 percentage points lower in Canada than in the United States (26.8% compared with 32.5%) and among women, it was more than 8 percentage points lower (24.5% compared with 33.7%).

According to CCHS self-reported data, obesity among Aboriginal people (excluding First Nations on-reserve) living both in the North (i.e., Yukon, Northwest Territories, and Nunavut) and in southern Canada has increased between 2000–2001 and 2005: in the North, from 20.2% to 25.4%, and in southern Canada, from 22.7% to 25.3%. However, only among North-residing Aboriginals ages 55 and older the difference over time was statistically significant. When the effects of age and sex were taken into account, the odds ratio of being obese was greater for Aboriginal people living in the North than for those in the south (Nolin *et al.*, 2004).

When comparisons were restricted to the non-Hispanic white population in each country, differences in obesity estimates were somewhat attenuated but the overall prevalence of obesity remained significantly lower in Canada compared with the United States. For instance, approximately 26% of the non-Hispanic white Canadian were obese compared with 33.0% of the non-Hispanic white population in the United States. Among the obese people with BMI in the outer limits the prevalence was fairly similar in the two countries (3.5% in Canada and about 5% in the United States).

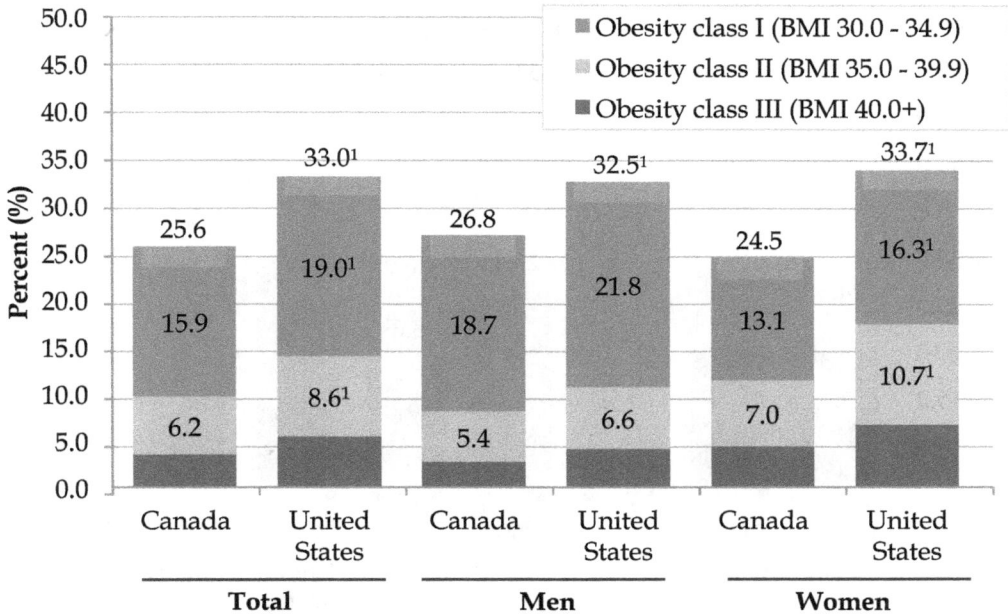

Figure 5: Prevalence of obesity among adults aged 20–79 years, by sex in Canada, 2007–2009, and United States, 2007–2008. Source: Center for Disease Control and Prevention; 1. Significantly different from estimate for Canada; 2. Use with caution (coefficient of variation 16.6% - 33.3%).

The racial makeup of the population in the two countries explains why the difference in prevalence is larger when the general populations are compared than when the non-Hispanic white populations are compared. In the United States, the minority population is mostly comprised of African American and Hispanic who have high prevalence of obesity than the non-Hispanic white population (Flegal *et al.*, 2010). Among nonwhite Canadians, the largest group is comprised of East/Southeast Asian peoples who have lower prevalence of obesity than the white population (Flegal *et al.*, 2010; Tremblay *et al.*, 2005).

5.1   Obesity Prevalence in the last 20 years in Canada and the United States

Current obesity prevalence estimates were compared with estimates from the 1988–1994 National Health & Nutrition Examination Survey (NHANES) and the 1986–1992 Canadian Heart Health Surveys (CHHS). In both countries the prevalence of obesity rose significantly since these earlier surveys, and the magnitude of the increases were fairly similar in the two countries (Figure 6 & 7). In Canadian men the prevalence rose by approximately 10 percentage points, and among American men the prevalence rose by 12 percentage points. Among women, the increase was approximately 8 percentage points in Canada and approximately 10 percentage points in the United States.

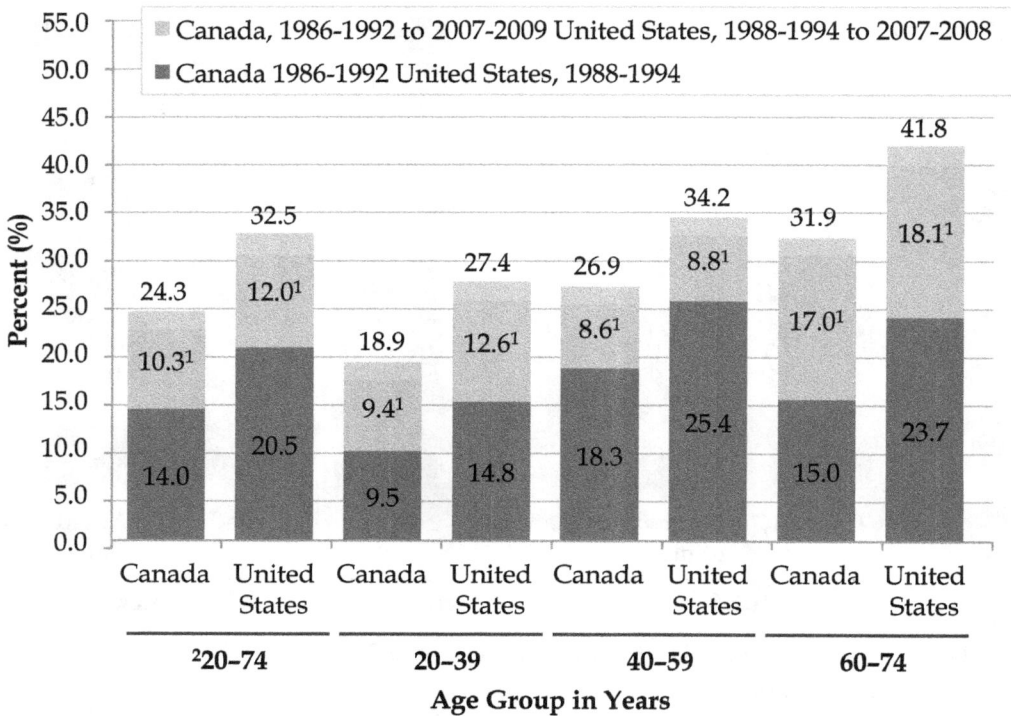

Figure 6: Prevalence of obesity in men aged 20–79 years, by age group in Canada, 1986–1992 and 2007–2009, and the United States, 1988–1994 and 2007–2008. Source: Center for Disease Control and Prevention; 1.Significantly different from 0 (p < 0.005); 2. Estimate age-standardized by the method to the 2000 United States Census population using age groups 20–39, 40–59, and 60–74.

5.2 Determinants of Obesity in Canada

Obesity is a significant population health concern. Research has shown that environmental, behavioral, social, cultural and genetic factors all contribute to the development of overweight and obesity. Obesity reduces life expectancy by more than 10 years as a comorbid illness with an increased risk of chronic conditions including diabetes, cancers, cardiovascular and musculoskeletal disease. Moreover, it is also related to impairment of the psychological well-being.

Populations who are moderately active or active in their leisure time are less likely to be obese. It has been shown that obese men consumed significantly more calories (2,820 versus 2,600 calories) as well contain higher percentages of total fat compared with non-obese men (Shields *et al.*, 2010; The Public Health Agency of Canada, 2011). The same is true for obese women; who tend to consume more calories (2,160 versus 1,970) than non-obese women.

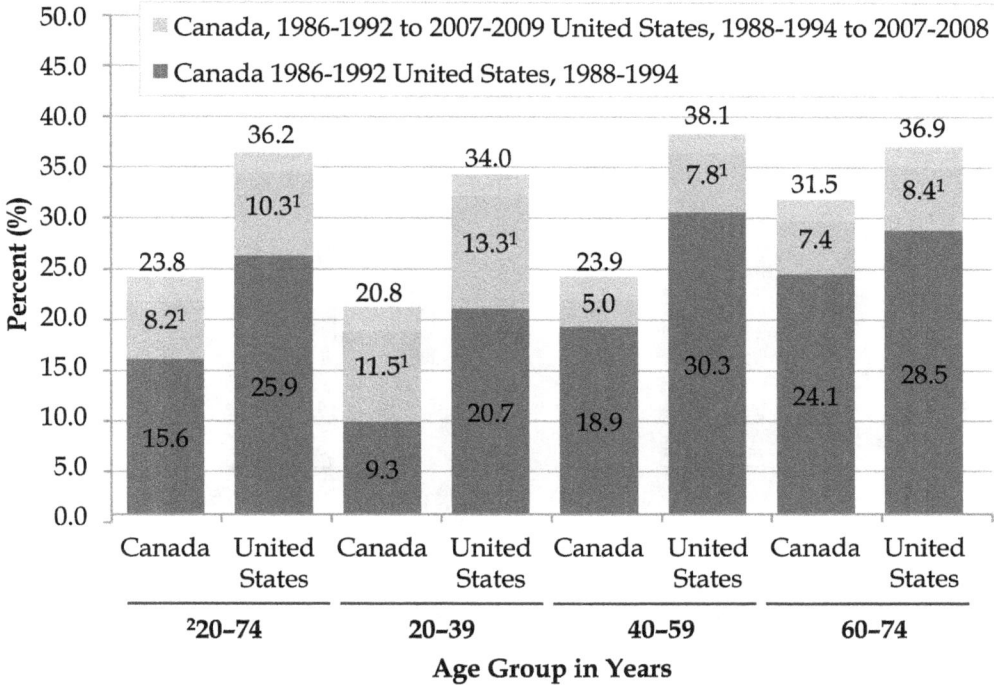

Figure 7: Prevalence of obesity in women aged 20–79 years, by age group in Canada, 1986–1992 and 2007–2009, and the United States, 1988–1994 and 2007–2008. Source: Center for Disease Control and Prevention; 1.Significantly different from 0 (p < 0.005); 2. Estimate age-standardized by the method to the 2000 United States Census population using age groups 20–39, 40–59, and 60–74

In addition to more proximal factors such as physical activity, sedentary behavior and diet which contribute to obesity there are several key distal factors that correlate with obesity including socioeconomic status, community, and environmental factors. Certain population groups have higher rates of obesity in Canada. These groups include Aboriginal peoples, many immigrant groups, those living in rural, remote areas, Atlantic region and, finally, those with a lower socio-economic status. Some of the of factors that are suspected to contribute to higher rates of obesity among marginalized populations include inequitable access to affordable, nutritious, safe, and culturally appropriate food and safe, adequate, and appropriate facilities for active recreation.

Analyses of the 2007/08 Canadian Community Health Survey (CCHS) propose that the relation between income and obesity varies by gender. As income increases obesity tends to decrease in women, however, similar pattern was not observed for men (Figure 8). In addition, among women but not in men, household income was associated with obesity. Marital status was found to be related to obesity among women, but not in men. Women, who were never married, widowed, separated or divorced, were more likely to be obese (Shields *et al.*, 2010; Statistics Canada, 2010; The Public Health Agency of Canada, 2011).

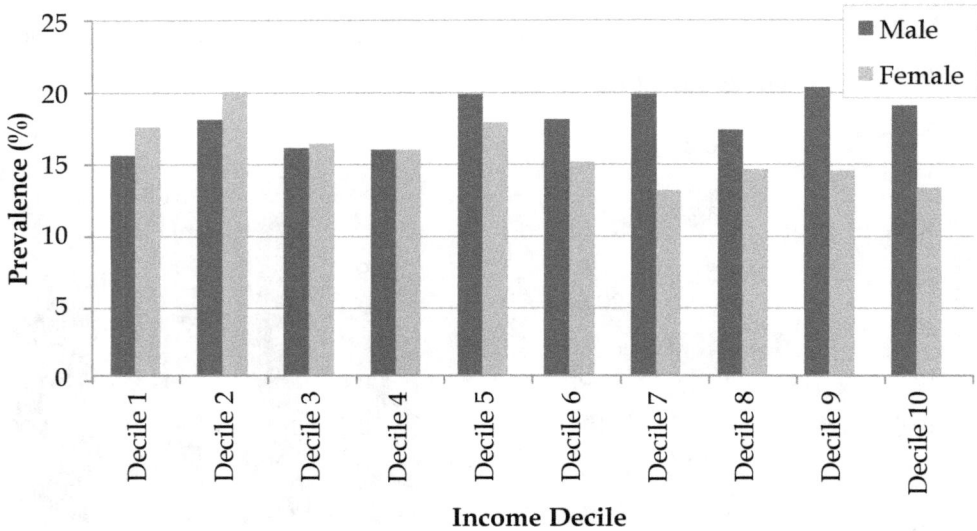

Figure 8: Prevalence of self-reported obesity among people eighteen years and older, by income decile, 2007. Source Public Health Agency of Canada. http://www.phac-aspc.gc.ca

Education has been shown to be associated with obesity, especially among men. An inverse pattern between education level and obesity prevalence has been observed for both men and women in the Canadian population. Men with secondary education or less are more likely to be obese than those who completed postgraduate education whereas the difference is less pronounced among women. For instance, the 2004 CCHS revealed that Canadian men with secondary education or less than secondary education have obesity rates of 32% and 35%, respectively compared with obesity rate of 22% in men with post-secondary education ($p < 0.05$).

The community-level factors such as neighborhood-level socioeconomic status correlate with obesity. The data from the 2005, 2007 and 2008 CCHS looked at disparities in obesity by socioeconomic status in Canada's Census Metropolitan Areas (CMAs). The analyses revealed that obesity was more prevalent in the most socioeconomically deprived areas than in the least deprived areas (The Public Health Agency of Canada, 2011). For instance, the obesity rates were 26% and 25% in the most socioeconomically deprived areas of Regina, Saskatchewan and Halifax, Nova Scotia, respectively compared with 14% and 11.2% in the highest socioeconomic status areas. There is also evidence of a relation between obesity and the community food environment and that relative availability of different types of food retailers around individuals' homes correlates with the bodyweight status of residents (Rosenheck, 2008; Pereira *et al.*, 2005; Spence *et al.*, 2009). The odds of being obese are related to diet and exercise. People who consume fruit and vegetables less frequently are more likely to be obese than those who eat such foods more often (Pérez, 2002). A Canadian study reported that lower the ratio of fast-food restaurants and convenience stores to grocery stores and product vendors near people's homes, the lower the odds of being obese (Spence *et al.*, 2009). Furthermore, community consumption of traditional foods has been associated with lower rates of obesity. The 2002/03 RHS reported that small First Nations communities which are more likely to consumed traditional foods had obesity rates of 25.7% compared with 44.2% in large communities (First Nations Centre, 2005).

6 Obesity and Economic Implication

There are currently few Canadian data on the long-term health impacts of obesity especially in children. Some studies focus on direct costs, while others examine indirect costs, or both (INSPQ, 2014). It has been estimated that obesity cost the Canadian economy approximately $4.6 billion in 2008, up $735 million or about 19% from $3.9 billion in 2000, based on costs associated with the eight chronic diseases most consistently linked to the obesity. Estimates rise to approximately $7.1 billion when it was based on the costs associated with 18 chronic diseases linked to the obesity (Aanis *et al.*, 2010; The Public Health Agency of Canada, 2011; Vanasse *et al.*, 2005). Of note, the economic impact of obesity is not confined to health service delivery. Productivity losses stemming from more widespread absenteeism and disability affect several economic sectors (INSPQ, 2014). Obesity influences physician cost that increases with age compared with normal weight persons. For example, 5.3% higher cost for obese young adults aged 18–39 years, 7.0% higher for obese middle-aged individuals aged 40–59 years and 28.3% higher for obese older adults aged 60 years or above (Janssen *et al.*, 2009).

6.1 Potential Interventions to Address Obesity

Obesity is not simply an issue of energy expenditure and intake, but rather is affected by a number of upstream factors that create the context in which people make decisions about physical activity and/or energy intake (Figure 9).

These contextual forces interact with underlying biological susceptibilities and often place eating and exercise behavior beyond an individual's rational control (Huang *et al.*, 2009). The causes of obesity are complex and multifaceted. These include not only individual choices but also environmental and social determinants. There has been an increasing focus on identification of potential risk factors and prevention and treatment strategies due to rising costs and poor health outcomes associated with obesity.

Different interventions in combination with a comprehensive prevention strategy at individual level can avoid up to 25, 000 deaths from chronic diseases every year resulting in 40, 000 years of life in good health (Dorothy, 2000; Roux & Donaldson, 2004). An organized program of counseling of obese people by their family doctors can also lead to an annual gain of 40,000 years of life in good health.

6.2 Cost-effectiveness of Prevention

Therapy for obesity either decrease energy intake or increase energy expenditure.

International Factors
- Globalization of Market
- Development
- Media

National Factors
- Transport
- Urbanization
- Health
- Social Security
- Media & Culture
- Education
- Food & Nutrition

Community/Locality
- Public Transport
- Publis Safety
- Health Care
- Sanitation
- Imported Food
- Agriculture/Local Market

Work/School/Home
- Access to Leisure Activity
- Labour
- Infections
- Word Food/ Activity
- Family & Home
- School Food/Activity

Individual
- Energy Expenditure
- Food Intake: Nutrient Density

Population

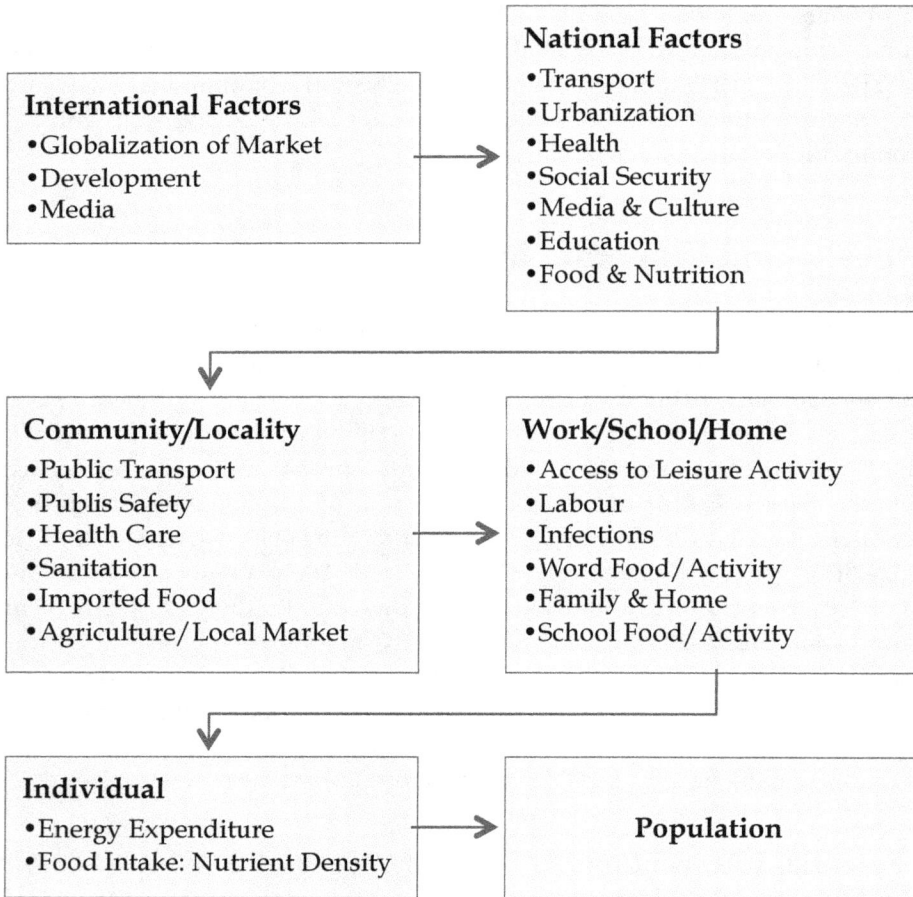

Figure 9: Obesity is caused by multiple factors that interact at various levels. Adopted from Huang TT, et al. Prev Chronic Dis 2009;6:A82.

Treatment includes behavior modification, dietary therapy, exercise, pharmacotherapy, liposuction, surgery and complementary therapies. Strategies aimed at preventing weight gain and obesity are vital and more cost effective than merely treating obesity once it has developed. Most prevention programs will cut health expenditures for chronic diseases and would cost less than CAD 200 million every year (Roux & Donaldson, 2004).

Prevention can promote health at a lower cost than many other treatments offered today by OECD health systems. In Canada, all of the prevention programs examined will be cost-effective in the long run — relative to the internationally accepted standard of around CAD 50, 000 per year of life gained in good health. Nevertheless, some programs will take a longer time to produce their health effects and therefore will be less cost-effective in the short run.

The costs of overweight or obesity may be grouped into two categories: direct and indirect costs. Direct costs are those for which payments are made, and indirect costs are those for which resources are lost (INSPQ, 2014). Direct costs include the cost of treatment, care and rehabilitation for illnesses associated with overweight or obesity (Figure 10). Indirect costs, referred to as "Negative Outputs/Welfare Losses," include reductions in economic productivity stemming from the poorer health, absenteeism, disability and premature mortality that are a result of overweight or obesity. Welfare losses, resulting from increased pain and suffering for example, are also considered indirect costs though they are rarely measured (Roux & Donaldson, 2004).

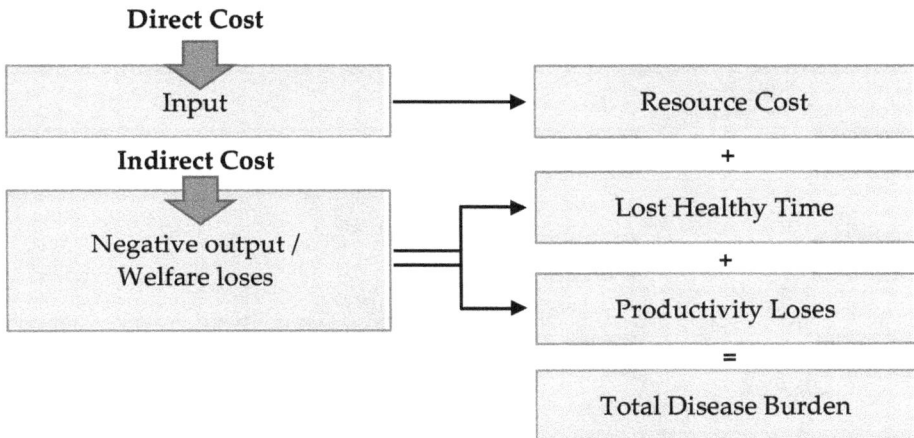

Figure 10: Obesity and overweight affect economy by direct (cost of treatment of illnesses associated with overweight or obesity) and indirect costs (Productivity losses, absenteeism and disability). Adopted from Roux and Donalds. Obes Res. 2004;12:173–9.

6.3   Strategies for Prevention

Obesity is a major challenge to the Canadian Society hence a combination of top-down and bottom-up approach is required to address it (Figure 11). A comprehensive, multi-sectoral response is required to reverse the rising prevalence of obesity in Canada.

Some key priority areas that require immediate attention in relationship with obesity are discussed below. The various approaches to deal with obesity are as follows:

- Research, surveillance and knowledge promotion

- Health services and clinical interventions that target individuals.

- Community-level interventions that directly influence individual and group behaviors.

- Public policies that target broad social or environmental determinants like government-level interventions including taxing unhealthy food, improving serving size, school level solution such as limiting access to unhealthy food.

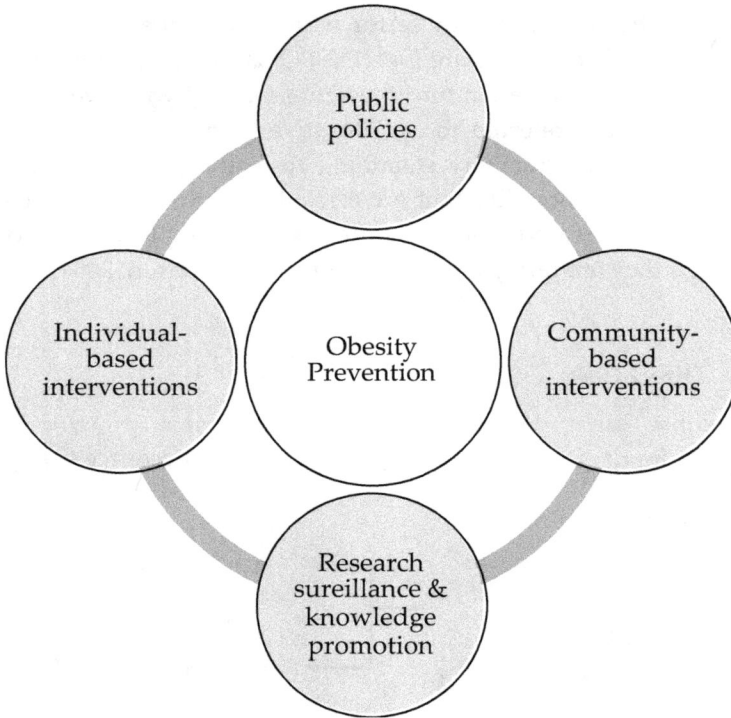

Figure 11: Strategies for Obesity Prevention.

7   Research, Surveillance & Knowledge Promotion

There have been concerns in the past about the availability of evidence and surveillance in relation to obesity in the Canada. With the recent release of new surveys like CHMS, more information is available for dissemination and intervention. However, there is a gap in the existing population-level data. It is important to identify and fill those gaps for effective surveillance and future prevention strategy. All the sources of data should be utilized to obtain important and useful information. Among those "administrative data" which is economical and plentiful is one of the key sources for future planning.

Developing and implementing effective interventions need better knowledge about various approaches that work in different settings with different populations as well as economic analyses to assess value for money. Social inequities, as a determinant of obesity, are a key priority area for research for effective preventative strategies. The lack of understanding about how socio- economic factors, such as poverty and income inequality, can act to increase the risk of obesity among certain marginalized groups. Furthermore, much of the research conducted on obesity and health in Canada is not producing policy-related data and information, thus limiting its usefulness to policy analysts and policy makers. It is vital to formulate existing and new data into a useable format which is accessible to policy makers. There is a need to increase funding for less traditional areas of policy-related research, such as historical research, research on values, and synthesis of research findings.

In light of the concerns raised over policy-related obesity research, development of a long-term data collection framework has been proposed. This framework will

- Review existing data sources and identify data gaps.

- Develop research which could assist policy makers to make informed decisions.

- Address relevant privacy issues research.

The collection of evidence on obesity and health should be identified as a priority area for action and research and action on obesity should be conducted side by side.

7.1   Individual-Based Interventions

The Canadian clinical practice guidelines for obesity provide recommendations regarding the prevention, screening and management of obesity in the clinical and community health settings (Lau *et al.*, 2007). These recommendations include education to encourage and support changes in behavior and attitudes; behavior modification training or therapy, including family-oriented behavior therapy for children; dietary interventions, such as an energy-reduced diet; regular physical activity in adults; and combined dietary and physical activity therapy among others (Lau *et al.*, 2007; Mendelson *et al.*, 2007; Prud'homme *et al.*, 2007; Vivienne *et al.*, 2007).

7.2   Community-Based Interventions

Community-based obesity prevention interventions include programs delivered in key settings such as workplaces and schools. A number of initiatives at the community level can be effective in influencing level of physical activity and healthy eating that are known to affect obesity.

7.2.1   Early Child Care and School Health

The foundation for lifelong good health is set in childhood. Hence, a life course approach to address factors influencing behavior and choices relating to balanced diets and physical activity is vital to tackle obesity. Early childhood is an important period for obesity prevention (Harvard School of Public Health). In 2002–2003, about 54% of Canadian children aged six months to five years were in some type of non-parental child care (Bushnik, 2006). Child care providers are in a unique position to educate parents about healthy eating and activity habits, and also to provide a healthy environment for children to eat, play, and grow.

Likewise, the school setting is a key location for health promotion within the community hub for the delivery of a variety of services and programs for all family members including provision of education on obesity related health risks, nutrition, and physical activity (Lagarde *et al.*, 2008). School-based prevention programs, without additional resources, can help students to eat better, be more active, and achieve healthier weights. Nutrition and physical activity lessons can be integrated in core curriculum including classroom subjects, physical education, and after-school programs. Schools can also promote health outside of the classroom, by surrounding students with opportunities to eat healthy and stay active. The optimal physical education program will foster a lifetime commitment to physical activity as part of a healthy lifestyle (American Heart Association, 2008).

7.2.2   Urban Design and Transportation: Healthy Activity Environment

An activity-friendly environment offers a variety of safe and affordable ways to be active thereby encourages physical activity (WHO, 2010). Community designs that discourage urban sprawl, prioritize recreation space, and facilitate safe walking and biking can increase everyday opportunities to be active (Harvard School of Public Health). Mixed-use development by allowing residential and commercial uses near each other, lowering the cost of sports programs or equipment, ensuring more equal access to recreation spaces and places are some interventions that can promote active transportation in a community. In addition crime- and violence-prevention measures to make neighborhoods feel safer is important to eliminate a major barrier to being active outdoors.

Inter-sectoral collaboration among transportation and city planners, private developers and employers, and community groups and educators is crucial for an activity-friendly environment to address obesity. Moreover, there should be further research on the relationship between urban design, transportation and physical planning and obesity for creation of best preventative strategies.

7.2.3   Food Secure Canada: Healthy Food Environment

Access to food is a fundamental human right (The universal declaration of human rights). The food environment includes features of the community, such as the number and kinds of food outlets in a neighborhood as well as consumer experience, such as the kinds of foods that are available, affordable, and of good quality (Story et al., 2008). Healthy food options may not readily be available, easily accessible, or affordable (Crawford et al., 2008, WHO, 2010). There is evidence that low-income and underserved communities often have limited access to stores that sell healthy food, especially high-quality fruits and vegetables. Furthermore rural communities often have a higher number of convenience stores, where healthy foods are less available than in larger, retail food markets (Liese et al., 2007).

Agriculture policy that focuses on increased planting and buying of fresh fruits and vegetables and revenue policy that focuses on increasing taxes on unhealthy foods and subsidizing the cost of healthy choices can promote healthy food environment. Local governments can use zoning regulations to address health and welfare of residents, who do not have access to healthy food by allowing designation of community food gardens and farmers markets and by limiting commercial food retail, such as fast food businesses. Communication policy can restrict advertisement on unhealthy foods. Improving transportation options to food sources such as supermarkets and farmers' markets by increasing bus routes or using supermarket-sponsored shuttle services can increase a community's access to healthy foods.

7.3   Public Policies

Collaboration among various levels of government and broad stakeholder consultations are required to balance environmental, economic, social and cultural needs and to coordinate community planning and design (Raine & Wilson, 2007). A number of public policy approaches can be undertaken to address obesity at the population level. These include land development, urban planning and transportation planning that promote active commuting and recreational physical activity; subsidy programs to support healthy eating (e.g. the Northern Fruit and Vegetable Pilot Programme in Ontario); financial incentives to promote physical activity (e.g., the Children's Fitness Tax Credit and the Federal Tax Credit for Public Transit); food labeling to help consumers understand the health implications of their choices; financial disincentives, such as a tax on "unhealthy" foods and beverages; and regulation of marketing to children, especially for energy-dense, nutrient-poor foods and beverages (He, 2009; Raine & Wilson, 2007; Tremblay, 2007; WHO, 2000).

8   Conclusions

There has been dramatic increase in prevalence of obesity, in Canada, over the last 30 years. This growing crisis is leading into a huge financial burden. The factors that lead to obesity are multifactorial and complex. Strategies aimed at preventing weight gain and obesity are vital than merely treating obesity once it has developed. Encouraging healthy weights will require multidisciplinary approach in all sectors and government level. Social, economic, environmental and physical factors must be incorporated in health policies and procedure to implement the change.

References

Aanis, A.H., Zhang, W., Bansback, N., et al. (2010). Obesity and overweight in Canada: an update. cost-of-illness study. Obesity Reviews. 11:31–40.

Aloia, J.F., Vaswani, A., Russo, L., et al. (1995). The influence of menopause and hormonal replacement therapy on body cell mass and body fat mass. Am J Obstet Gynecol. 172:896.

American Heart Association. (2008). Policy Position Statement on Physical Education in Schools. http://www.heart.org/idc/groups/heart-public/@wcm/@adv/documents/downloadable/ucm_301654.pdf (accessed September 2014)

Nolin, B., Lamontagne L., & Tremblay, A. (2004). Nunavik Iinuit Health Survey 2004, Quanuipptaa? How are we? Physical Activity, Anthropometry and Perception of Body

Weight (Québec.: Nunavik Regional Board of Health and Social Services, 2007).

Bray, G.A. & Bellanger, T. (2006). Epidemiology, trends, and morbidities of obesity and the metabolic syndrome. Endocrine. 29:109.

Bushnik, T. (2006). Child Care in Canada. Statistic Canada. http://publications.gc.ca/Collection/Statcan/89-599-MIE/89-599-MIE2006003.pdf (accessed September 2014)

Christakis, N.A. & Fowler, J.H. (2007). The spread of obesity in a large social network over 32 years. N Engl J Med. 357:370.

Crawford, D., Timperio, A.F., Salmon, J.A., et al. (2008). Neighborhood fast food outlets and obesity in children and adults: the CLAN Study. Int J Pediatr Obes. 3:249–256.

Dorothy, P. (2000). Rice Cost of Illness Studies: What Is Good About Them. Injury Prevention. 6:177.

Elgar, F. & Stewart, J. (2008). Validity of Self-Report Screening for Overweight and Obesity. Evidence from the Canadian Community Health Survey. Can J Public Health. 99:423–427.

Field, A.E., Coakley, E.H., Must, A., Spadano, J.L., Laird, N., Dietz, W.H., Rimm, E. & Colditz, G.A. (2001). Impact of overweight on the risk of developing common chronic diseases during a 10-year period. Arch Intern Med. 161:1581–1586.

First Nations Centre. (2005). First Nations Regional Longitudinal Health Survey (RHS) 2002/03, Results for Adults, Youth and Children Living in First Nations Communities (Ottawa, Ont.: RHS, 2007). http://fnigc.ca/sites/default/files/ENpdf/RHS_2002/rhs2002-03-technical_report.pdf (accessed April 14th 2014)

Flegal, K.M., Carroll, M.D., Ogden, C.L. & Curtin, L.R. (2010). Prevalence and trends in obesity among US adults, 1999–2008. JAMA. 303:235–41.

Flegal, K.M., Troiano, R.P., Pamuk, E.R., et al. (1995). The influence of smoking cessation on the prevalence of overweight in the United States. N Engl J Med. 333:1165.

Gillman, M.W., Rifas-Shiman, S.L., Camargo, C.A. Jr, et al. (2001). Risk of overweight among adolescents who were breastfed as infants. JAMA. 285:2461.

Harvard School of Public Health. Obesity prevention strategies. http://www.hsph.harvard.edu/obesity-prevention-source/obesity-prevention/early-child-care/early-child-care-obesity-prevention-recommendation-complete-list/ (accessed Septem-ber 2014)

He, M., Beynon, C. & Sanster, M., et al. (2009). Impact Evaluation of the Northern Fruit and Vegetable Pilot Programme — a Cluster-Randomised Controlled Trial. Public Health Nutr. 12:2199–2208.

Hediger, M.L., Overpeck, M.D., Kuczmarski, R.J. & Ruan, W.J. (2001). Association between infant breastfeeding and overweight in young children. JAMA. 285:2453.

Hochberg, I. & Hochberg, Z. (2010). Expanding the definition of hypothalamic obesity. Obes Rev. 11:709.

Huang, T.T., Drewnowski, A., Kumanyika, S.K. & Glass, T.A. (2009). A systems-oriented multi-level framework for addressing obesity in the 21st century. Prev Chronic Dis. 6:A82

INSPQ. (2014). *The economic impact of obesity and overweight http://www.inspq.qc.ca/pdf/ publications/1799_Topo_9_VA.pdf*

Janssen, I., Lam, M. & Katzmarzyk, P.T. (2009). *Influence of Overweight and Obesity on Physician Costs in Adolescents and Adults in Ontario, Canada. Obesity Reviews. 10:51–57.*

Knudsen, N., Laurberg, P., Rasmussen, L.B., et al. (2005). *Small differences in thyroid function may be important for body mass index and the occurrence of obesity in the population. J Clin Endocrinol Metab. 90:4019.*

Lagarde, F., LeBlanc, C.M.A., McKenna, M., et al. (2008). *School policy framework: implementation of the WHO global strategy on diet, physical activity and health Geneva, Switzerland: World Health Organization.*

Lau David, C.W. et al. (2007). *2006 Canadian clinical practice guidelines on the management and prevention of obesity in adults and children. CMAJ. 176(8 suppl):1–117.*

Lawson, O.J., Williamson, D.A., Champagne, C.M., et al. (1995). *The association of body weight, dietary intake, and energy expenditure with dietary restraint and disinhibition. Obes Res. 3:153.*

Leslie, W.S., Hankey, C.R. & Lean, M.E. (2007). *Weight gain as an adverse effect of some commonly prescribed drugs: a systematic review. QJM. 100:395.*

Liese, A.D., Weis, K.E., Pluto, D., et al. (2007). *Food store types, availability and cost of foods in a rural environment. J Am Dietetic Assoc. 107:1916–23.*

Lix, L.M., Bruce, S., Sarkar, J. & Young, T.K. (2009). *Risk Factors and Chronic Conditions Among Aboriginal and Non-Aboriginal Populations. Health Rep 2009;20:21–29.*

Lukanova, A., Bjor, O., Kaaks, R., Lenner, P., Lindahl, B., Hallmans, G. & Stattin, P. (2006). *Body mass index and cancer: results from the Northern Sweden Health and Disease Cohort. Int J Cancer. 118:458–466.*

Shields, M., et al. (2010). *Fitness of Canadian Adults: Results from the 2007–2009 Canadian Health Measures Survey. Health Rep. 21:1–15.*

Mendelson, R., Martino, R., Clarke, C., et al. (2007). *Dietary Interventions for the Treatment of Obesity in Adults. CMAJ.176 (8 suppl):57–59.*

Mozaffarian, D., Hao, T., Rimm, E.B., et al. (2011) *Changes in diet and lifestyle and long-term weight gain in women and men. N Engl J Med. 364:2392.*

Must, A., Spadano, J., Coakley, E.H., Field, A.E., et al. (1999). *The disease burden associated with overweight and obesity. JAMA. 282:1523–1529.*

National Institutes of Health. National Heart, Lung, and Blood Institute. (1998). *Clinical guidelines on the identification, evaluation, and treatment of overweight and obesity in adults: The evidence report. Obes Res. 6 Suppl 2:515.*

OECD. *Health policies and data. http://www.oecd.org/home. (accessed April 2014)*

Pereira, M.A., Kartashov, A.I., Ebbeling, C.B., et al. (2005). *Fast-food habits, weight gain, and insulin resistance (the CARDIA study): 15-year prospective analysis. Lancet. 365:36–42*

Pérez, C.E. (2002). *Fruit and vegetable consumption. Health Reports (Statistics Canada, Catalogue 82-003). 13:23–31.*

Pi-Sunyer, F.X. (1993). *Medical hazards of obesity. Ann Intern Med 1993; 119:655–660.*

Power, C. & Jefferis, B.J. (2002). *Fetal environment and subsequent obesity: a study of maternal smoking. Int J Epidemiol. 31:413.*

Prud'homme, D., Doucet, E., Dionne, I. & Ross, R. (2007). *Physical Activity and Exercise Therapy — Adults. CMAJ. 176 (8 suppl):e-64–66.*

Raine, K., & Wilson, E. (2007). *Obesity Prevention in the Canadian Population: Policy Recommendations for Environmental Change. CMAJ. 176 (8 suppl):106–112.*

Rosenheck, R. (2008). *Fast food consumption and increased caloric intake: A systematic review of a trajectory towards weight gain and obesity risk. Obes Rev. 9:535–547.*

Roux, L. & Donaldson, C. (2004). *Economics and obesity: costing the problem or evaluating solutions? Obes Res. 12:173–9.*

Spence, J., Cutumisu, N., Edwards, J., et al. (2009). *Relation Between Local Food Environments and Obesity Among Adults. BMC Public Health. 9:192.*

Spiegel, K., Tasali, E., Penev, P. & Van Cauter, E. (2004). *Brief communication: Sleep curtailment in healthy young men is associated with decreased leptin levels, elevated ghrelin levels, and increased hunger and appetite. Ann Intern Med. 141:846.*

Statistics Canada. (2009). *Aboriginal Peoples Survey - Concepts and Methods Guide (Ottawa, Ont.: Statistics Canada, 2009). http://www.statcan.gc.ca/pub/89-637-x/89-637-x2008003-eng.htm (accessed April 5th 2014).*

Statistics Canada. (2010). *Canadian Health Measures Survey: Cycle 1 Data Tables: Introduction (Ottawa, Ont.: Statistics Canada, 2010). http://www.statcan.gc.ca/pub/82-623-x/2010001/part-partie1-eng.htm (accessed March 13th 2014)*

Story, M., Kaphingst, K.M., Robinson-O'Brien, R. & Glanz, K. (2008). *Creating healthy food and eating environments: policy and environmental approaches. Annu Rev Public Health. 29:253–72.*

The, N.S., Suchindran, C., North, K.E., et al. (2010). *Association of adolescent obesity with risk of severe obesity in adulthood. JAMA. 304:2042.*

The Public Health Agency of Canada. (2011). *http://www.phac-aspc.gc.ca/hp-ps/hl-mvs/oic-oac/assets/pdf/oic-oac-eng.pdf (accessed March 2nd 2014)*

The universal declaration of human rights *http://www.un.org/en/documents/udhr/index (accessed September 2014)*

Tremblay, M.S., Pérez, C.E., Ardern, C.I., Bryan, S.N. & Katzmarzyk, P.T. (2005). *Obesity, overweight and ethnicity. Statistics Canada, Catalogue 82–003. Health Rep. 16:23–34.*

Tremblay, M. (2007). *Major Initiatives Related to Childhood Obesity and Physical Inactivity in Canada. The Year in Review. Can J Public Health. 98:457–459.*

Vanasse, A., Demeres, M., Hemiari & A., et al. (2005). *Obesity in Canada: Where and How*

Many? Int J Obes. 30:677–683.

Vasan, R.S., Pencina, M.J., Cobain, M., et al. (2005). Estimated risks for developing obesity in the Framingham Heart Study. Ann Intern Med.143:473.

Visscher, T.L. & Seidell, J.C. (2001). The public health impact of obesity. Annu. Rev. Public Health. 22:355–375.

Vivienne, A. V., Hanning, R. & McCargar, L.. (2007). Combined Diet and Exercise in the Treatment of Pediatric Overweight and Obesity. CMAJ.176 (8 suppl):87–88.

Whitaker, R.C., Wright, J.A., Pepe, M.S., et al. (1997). Predicting obesity in young adulthood from childhood and parental obesity. N Engl J Med. 337:869.

WHO. (1998). WHO Consultation on Obesity. Obesity: Preventing and managing the global epidemic. Geneva, 3–5 June 1997. World Health Organization, Geneva. http://whqlibdoc. who.int/hq/1998/WHO_NUT_NCD_98.1_(p1–158).pdf (accessed March 14th 2014).

WHO. (2000). Preventing and Managing the Global Epidemic. WHO Technical Report Series 894. http://whqlibdoc.who.int/trs/WHO_TRS_894.pdf (accessed September 2014)

WHO. (2010). Global recommendation on physical activity for health. Geneva, Switzerland: World Health Organization; 2010. http://whqlibdoc.who.int/publications/2010/ 9789241599979_eng.pdf (accessed September 2014)

Chapter 2

Environmental Changes as Part of Multi-component School-based Obesity Prevention Interventions: A Systematic Qualitative Review

Melinda Ickes[1], Jennifer McMullen[1], Manoj Sharma[2]

1 Introduction

Childhood obesity continues to threaten health outcomes and quality of life world-wide. By 2020, the prevalence of childhood obesity is projected to increase from 6.7% to 9.1% (Onis *et al.*, 2010). Although obesity continues to be a global concern, prevalence rates in the United States tend to be higher as compared to other developed countries, with 16.9% of 2–19 year olds obese and 31.7% overweight or obese (Fryar *et al.*, 2010; Ogden *et al.*, 2012;Olds *et al.*, 2011), reinforcing the need to target school-aged children. Recent findings indicate a plateau in the spiked prevalence increases observed over the past 30 years, and in some cases, a marked decline in several developed countries, though rates remain unacceptably high (Olds *et al.*, 2011). As a result, the need to determine effective population-based strategies to prevent and mitigate childhood overweight and obesity still remains a global priority.

The health, social, and economic consequences related to obesity cannot be ignored (Freedman *et al.*, 2007; French *et al.*, 1995; Whitlock *et al.*, 2005; Withrow & Alter, 2011). Childhood obesity has been associated with a number of adverse secondary health-related outcomes, including increased blood pressure and increased cholesterol levels (Freedman *et al.*, 2007) and increased risk of diabetes mellitus type 2 (Whitlock *et*

[1] Department of Kinesiology and Health Promotion, University of Kentucky, USA
[2] Behavioral & Environmental Health, Jackson State University, United States

al., 2005). Negative psychological emotional outcomes have also been reported, including low self-esteem and depression (French *et al.*, 1995). There is stigma related to being overweight and obese, which may decreases a person's quality of life (French *et al.*, 1995). Studies suggest that obese children are more likely to become obese adults, further bringing to attention the need to prioritize preventative measures which reach the majority of school-aged children (Freedman *et al.*, 2007).

Determinants of obesity may be influenced by the following: genetics, socioeconomic status, conditions within the first year of life, maternal behaviors, family food environment and subsequent dietary behaviors, participation in physical activity, a sedentary lifestyle, and environmental factors that impact one's accessibility to healthy food and physical activity (Budd *et al.*, 2006; Rennie *et al.*, 2005; Robert Wood Johnson Foundation [RWJF], 2013; Sharma & Ickes, 2008; Young *et al.*, 2012). Specifically, environmental factors may be broken down into the following types: physical (what is available), economic (associated costs), political (policies and regulations), and sociocultural (attitudes and beliefs) (Summerbell *et al.*, 2005). Research lends support to the idea that one of the most important environmental determinants linked to obesity is a child's school. Access to nutritious foods, mandated physical education, nutrition and physical activity concepts integrated into the curriculum, and related school wellness policies are a few examples of how the school environment may play a role in childhood overweight and/or obesity (Sharma & Ickes, 2008). As a result, targeting childhood obesity programs at schools, can truly impact this global epidemic (Summerbell *et al.*, 2005). Perhaps, in part, because of the previous focus on nutrition and physical activity at the individual level, school-based obesity programs have not consistently resulted in the success one might expect (The Community Guide, n.d.). This provides rationale for incorporating interventions which look beyond the individual level and include broader environmental changes.

School-based programs have historically been used to impact child health and constitute an important strategy in public health. Specifically, preventive efforts targeting childhood obesity have frequently focused on schools as an important setting, though their long-term success has been limited (RWJF, 2013; Sharma & Ickes, 2008). Schools are considered an ideal target, given the capability to prevent obesity through the promotion of physical activity, nutritious food offerings, and nutrition education through practice, policy, and supportive environments. Students consume 25% to 33% of their daily energy (Farris *et al.*, 1992) and amass 20% to 30% of daily physical activity at school, supporting the potential impact that schools can have in affecting students' health by improving the related environment (Myers *et al.*, 1996; Ross & Gilbert, 1985). Past systematic reviews report conflicting results on the short- and long-term success of school-based obesity prevention interventions (Sharma, 2006, 2007; Sharma & Ickes, 2008; Summerbell *et al.*, 2005). However, little is known about the specific impact environmental strategies can have when integrated into school-based interventions. Although there is evidence to support environmental approaches as part of school-based interventions (French *et al.*, 2001; Sallis *et al.*, 1995), environmental and policy interventions are the least studied component of school health promotion. Thus, the effectiveness should be further investigated to bring to light strategies that could increase the efficacy of school-based obesity prevention interventions Therefore, the purpose of this chapter is to synthesize school-based obesity prevention interventions which incorporate environmental change and provide recommendations for the development of future interventions.

2. Experimental

2.1   Methods

2.1.1   Inclusion/Exclusion Criteria

Inclusion criteria for this review included (1) primary research; (2) overweight or obesity prevention interventions; (3) school-based; (4) studies that were published between January 1, 2002 – July 1, 2014 within select databases; (5) published in the English language; (6) child-based programs, which could include parents; (7) outcome-based (i.e., presentation of results beyond process evaluation and baseline characteristics); and (8) incorporated environmental change(s) as at least one intervention strategy. Interventions implemented in pre-schools, early childcare programs, or after-school programs were excluded. In this review, primary research was defined as including studies which were carried out to acquire the data first-hand, rather than being gathered from previously used sources. Additionally, school-based was defined as an intervention which was implemented during regular school hours for children in kindergarten through senior year of high school and/or primary through secondary grades as defined internationally. Lastly, the Analysis Grid for Environments Linked to Obesity (ANGELO) framework was used to classify the various environmental determinants. The ANGELO framework dissects the environment by type: physical (what is available), economic (associated costs), political (the rules) and sociocultural (attitudes and beliefs) (Summerbell et al., 2005). For the purpose of this study, environmental changes were operationalized to include physical and political factors (e.g., nutrition and physical activity integrated into the curriculum, making healthy foods available, etc.).

2.1.2   Study Abstraction

Two researchers conducted an extensive independent literature search in order to incorporate all pertinent studies in this review. Searches were conducted utilizing the following databases: Academic Search Premier, CINAHL (Cumulative Index to Nursing and Allied Health), MEDLINE (Medical Literature Analysis and Retrieval System Online), ERIC (Education Resources Information Center), and Psychology and Behavioral Sciences Collection. The following keywords were used: [obese OR overweight] AND [school OR school-based] AND [youth OR child OR adolescent] AND [prevention OR intervention OR treatment OR program OR study]. Limits of scholarly journals (peer-reviewed) were set. A total of 12,294 documents were found using the aforementioned criteria. Articles were then further reduced based on inclusion and exclusion criteria, including that interventions had at least one environmental component. See Figure 1 for a flow diagram. In addition, a thorough assessment of all references cited from the articles identified in the search was conducted to uncover any publications that did not surface during the initial search process, resulting in one additional intervention to include (Singh *et al.*, 2007). Additionally, a final review of all references from manuscripts included in this study was conducted, resulting in three additional interventions appropriate for inclusion. Thus, a total of 15 interventions were included in this review.

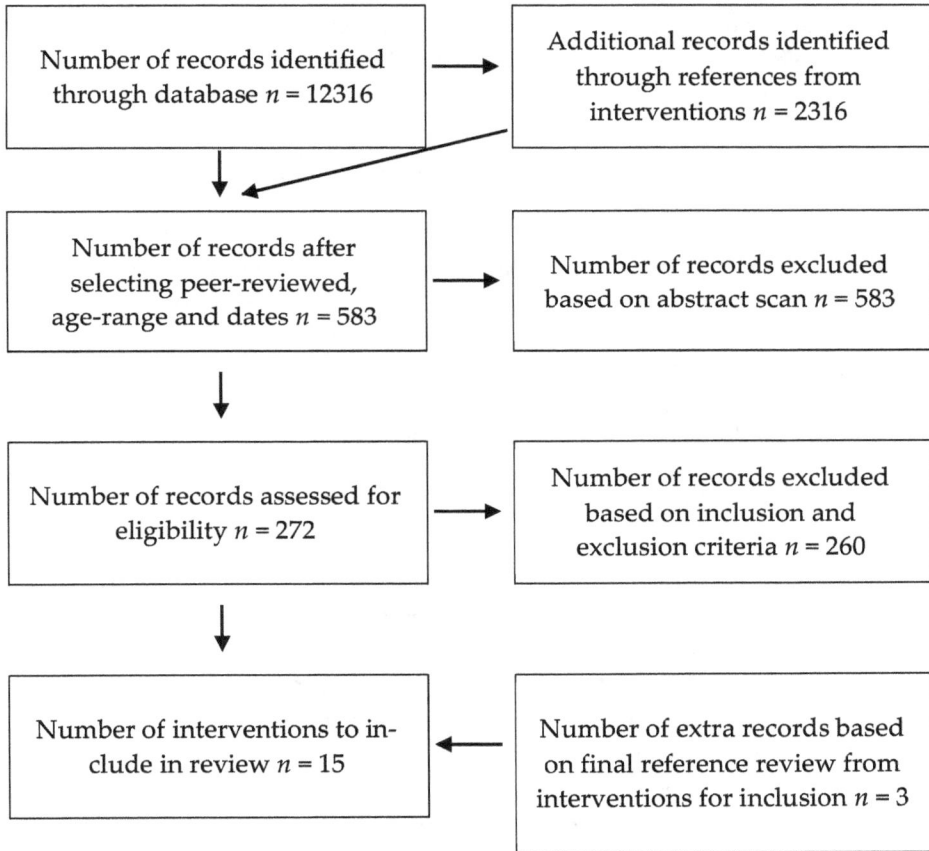

Figure 1. Summary of search results.

2.2   Data Extraction

Data from the studies were extracted, independently, by two researchers using a standardized form that the researchers created. Discrepancies were examined by all three authors and non-disputed data recorded. There was no instance of disagreement with regards to studies meeting inclusion criteria. Extracted data included: author, publication year, participant data, environmental change operationalized, additional strategies utilized, theory used, research design, outcomes, interventions dosage and duration and salient findings.

3   Results and Discussion

3.1   Sample and Design

The review was limited to interventions which took place in a school-based environment. Of the interventions, forty percent ($n = 6$) took place in the United States (Donnelly et al., 2008; Foster et al., 2008; Hollar et al., 2010; Johnston et al., 2013; Sallis et al., 2003; Wang et al., 2010) and sixty percent ($n = 9$) were imple mented outside of the United States. Overall, 80% ($n = 12$) of the interventions took place at the elementary school level. Three of the interventions focused on middle school settings (Haernes et al., 2006; Sallis et al., 2003; Singh et al., 2007).

Of the included interventions, 47% ($n = 7$) specifically targeted low-income schools. The number of participants within the interventions varied significantly, ranging from 168 participants (Lopes et al., 2009), to one study which enrolled 24 schools, each with mean enrollment of 1109 students (Sallis et al., 2003). There were three types of study designs utilized throughout the interventions. The most common design was randomized controlled trial ($n = 10$, 67). The second most frequent design was quasi-experimental ($n = 4$, 33%). Additionally, one study utilized a prospective design (Wang et al., 2010).

3.2   Theoretical Framework

Use of theory was mentioned in 20% ($n = 3$) of the interventions (Graf et al., 2008; Haernes et al., 2006; Muckelbauer et al., 2009), all of which were implemented internationally. All interventions used the Theory of Planned Behavior (TPB), while one additionally utilized the Transtheoretical Model (TTM). Two of the interventions did not detail how the theory was operationalized nor did they measure the changes in constructs of the theory before and after the interventions. However, one intervention mentioned that normative feedback, based on questionnaire completion, was given based upon the selected theoretical constructs (Haernes et al., 2006).

3.3   Intervention Approach

Duration of the interventions ranged from two weeks ($n = 1$) to four years ($n = 1$). The majority of interventions were implemented two years or more ($n = 9$, 60%). Dosage of the interventions varied from daily to weekly sessions. Of the included interventions, 53% ($n = 8$) of the interventions took place daily, 33% ($n = 4$) took place weekly or more than once throughout the week, and one intervention implemented both weekly and daily regularly occurring intervention strategies (Graf et al., 2008). One intervention did not mention a specific dosage, but said that the strategies occurred over the course of the year (Foster *et al.*, 2008). Another study said its intervention occurred over two fixed periods throughout the year, with no further specification given (Singh *et al.*, 2007).

A variety of environmental strategies were utilized throughout the included interventions. Strategies included: implementation of school nutrition policy and physical activity policy, nutrition and healthy lifestyle curricula, development and utilization of school gardens (Hollar *et al.*, 2010), instillation of water fountains (Muckelbauer *et al.*, 2009) and school-based cooking classes (Hollar *et al.*, 2010; Johnston *et al.*, 2013; Wang *et al.*, 2010). Four interventions (27%) explicitly mentioned the use of both nutrition education and physical education/activity components as environmental intervention strategies (Graf *et al.*, 2008; Haernes *et al.*, 2006; Hollar *et al.*, 2010; Sallis *et al.*, 2003). Four interventions (27%) focused solely on nutrition changes and education (Foster *et al.*, 2008; Johnston *et al.*, 2013; Muckelbauer *et al.*, 2009; Wang *et al.*, 2010), while five (33%) focused exclusively on physical activity changes (Donnelly *et al.*, 2009; Lopes *et al.*, 2009; Ploeg *et al.*, 2014; Sacchetti *et al.*, 2013). Additionally, two interventions focused on physical activity changes as well as changes to the curriculum regarding health, biology, and PE (Graf *et al.*, 2005; Singh *et al.*, 2007). Of the interventions that included nutrition-focused environmental strategies, four of the six specifically implemented policy and/or curricula change. Of those that focused on physical activity-related environmental changes, seven interventions specifically implemented policy and/or curricula change. Among the interventions that utilized a nutritional education component, four (27%) explicitly mentioned the use of hands-on nutritional activities such as school gardens, cooking classes, and computer-tailored intervention for nutrition. All of the interventions integrated other strategies in conjunction with environmental changes. Other strategies included school self-assessment and social marketing (Foster *et al.*, 2008), increasing daily physical activity (Donnelly *et al.*, 2009; Graf *et al.*, 2008; Haernes *et al.*, 2006; Hartman *et al.*, 2010; Pleg *et al.*, 2014; Sacchetti *et al.*, 2013; Sallis *et al.*, 2003), adding physical activity-related games and activities to the playground and classroom (Sacchetti *et al.*, 2013), maintaining food diaries/logs (Ploeg *et al.*, 2014; Swinburn *et al.*, 1999), and tracking physical activity with pedometers (Ploeg *et al.*, 2014). Nine of the studies (60%) employed a parental component, all of which had statistically significant findings. These interventions had varying degrees of parental involvement ranging from phone calls, parent teacher association (PTA) meetings, and newsletters sent home to reinforce changes implemented in the school. None of the studies specifically mentioned cultural relevance.

3.4   Intervention Outcomes and Measures

All of the interventions provided outcome data, although the primary outcomes varied. Body mass index (BMI) and/or overweight or obesity was the primary outcome for the majority of interventions (80%, $n = 12$). Overall, all but one of the interventions (Graf *et al.*, 2008) measuring BMI reported a decrease in BMI and/or overweight or obesity measures, ten of which were statistically significant. The other three studies did not measure BMI, but instead, psychosocial quality of life (Hartmann *et al.*, 2010), participation in moderate and vigorous physical activity (Lopes *et al.*, 2009), and increase in consumption of and preference for fruits and vegetables (Wang *et al.*, 2010), all of which resulted in improvements from pre-to post-intervention. Additionally, lateral jumping and a 6-minute run were primary outcomes for one intervention, both of which resulted in statistically significant findings for the intervention group (Graf *et al.*, 2008). All of the interventions reported positive changes related to at least one of their identified primary outcomes. Fourteen of the interventions (93%) resulted in at least one statistically significant finding.

Of the included interventions, 33% (*n* = 5) followed-up with participants post-intervention (Graf *et al.*, 2005, 2008; Johnston *et al.*, 2013; Muckelbauer *et al.*, 2009; Sacchetti *et al.*, 2013), but the findings from such follow-ups varied. Of the four interventions that explicitly mentioned the follow-up results, three noted positive findings, including significantly lower increase in BMI and/or risk of overweight (Haernes *et al.*, 2006; Muckelbauer *et al.*, 2009; Sacchetti *et al.*, 2013).

4 Discussion

The purpose of this study was to synthesize school-based obesity prevention interventions which incorporated environmental changes and provide recommendations for the development of future interventions. Over a 12 ½ year timeframe, 15 interventions incorporated environmental change as part of a school-based obesity prevention intervention. Considering the growing evidence and support for environmental changes as an integral component to obesity prevention (Sallis *et al.*, 1995), there are considerably more school-based interventions with an environmental component included in this review as compared to those included in previous reviews of this kind (Sharma, 2006; Sharma & Ickes, 2008; The Community Guide, n.d.). The positive, health-enhancing outcomes from the studies included in this review reinforce the need for further research on school-based obesity prevention interventions linked to environmental strategies.

Overall, findings from the included interventions were promising, with each resulting in at least one positive, measurable outcome. The majority of the interventions took place at the elementary school level. Elementary schools appear to be an ideal setting for the implementation of obesity prevention interventions given the opportunities for promoting both physical activity and nutrition behaviors (RWFJ, 2013). Elementary schools may have more flexibility within the classroom to integrate curriculum changes, increase physical activity during the school day, and alter the school environment (Sharma, 2006; Sharma & Ickes, 2008; Summerbell *et al.*, 2005). Also elementary school age is conducive to individual level behavior change strategies which can be dovetailed with successful environmental strategies. There remains, however, a need for future interventions utilizing similar environmental strategies to target middle and high school-aged children .Although numerous studies suggest that it is easier to influence behaviors at a younger age, the likelihood that obesity will exist beyond adolescence rises as at-risk individuals enter adulthood without intervention (Freedman *et al.*, 2007).

Author, Year	Sample Description	Sample Size	Research Design	Dosage and Duration	Environmental Intervention Strategies
Donnelly et al. 2009	U.S.; ELEM; low-income; BL BMI Int = 17.9 ± 3.1; Cnt = 18.0 ± 3.7	N = 1527; Int = 814; Cnt = 713	RCT	90 min/week of physically active academic lessons; 3 years	Lessons from Take 10![®], PA incorporated across all content areas
Foster et al. 2008	U.S.; low-income; BL OW = 17%; BL OB = 22-25%	N = 1349; Int = 749; Cnt = 600	RCT	50 h/year; 2 years	PC; School self assessment, nutrition education, nutrition policy, social marketing
Graf et al. 2005	International; ELEM; BL BMI Mean = 16.3; Range = 16.2 - 28	N = 651; Int = 460; Cnt = 191	RCT	Daily PA and weekly Health Ed; 2 years	Increased daily PA, improved Health Ed Curriculum
Graf et al. 2008	International; ELEM; BL OW = 8.1%; BL OB = 6.6%	N = 611; Cnt = 178; Int = 433	Quasi-experimental	Extra health lesson/week (20 - 30 min), and one 5 min PA break/morning; 4 years	PC; extra health lesson weekly, mini PA breaks daily
Haernes et al. 2006	International; MS; BL Mean BMI Int w/ PC = 19.7 ± 3.8; Int = 19.5 ± 3.5; Cnt 19 ± 3.5	BL N = 2840; Int w/ PC = 1226; Int alone = 1006; Cnt = 759	RCT	Daily PA and nutrition offerings; 2 years	Increased daily PA, computer tailored intervention for PA and nutrition, food intervention including increased daily fruit distribution

Continued on next page....

...Continued from previous pages

Author, Year	Sample Description	Sample Size	Research Design	Dosage and Duration	Environmental Intervention Strategies
Hartmann et al. 2010	International; ELEM; BL OW and/or OB: 1st grade Cnt = 25%; 1st grade Int = 26%; 5th grade Cnt = 26%; 5th grade Int = 25%	N = 411; 1st grade Cnt = 69; 1st grade Int = 111; 5th grade Cnt = 85; 5th grade Int	RCT	Daily PE, short activity breaks/day during lessons; 1 year	PC; Increased PA, playground changes, PA homework
Hollar et al. 2010	U.S.; ELEM; Low-income; BL OW Int = 7.3%; Cnt = 8.5%; BL OB Int = 17.6%; Cnt = 22.9%	N = 1173; Int = 974, Cnt = 199	Quasi-experimental	Monthly nutritional activities, 10 – 15 min PA/day; 2 years	USDA-NSLP school-provided meals, nutrition and healthy lifestyle curricula, monthly activities, mandated PA breaks, structured PE activities
Johnston et al. 2013	U.S.; ELEM; BL OW/OB = 33%	N = 835; Int PFI (professional facilitated information): N = 509 Int SH (self-help): N = 326	RCT	5 teaching moments/week, 1 lesson/week, 1 activity/2 weeks, and 1 school-wide activity/semester; 2 years	PC; Healthy lessons incorporated into main subject areas in accordance with state curriculum

Continued on next page...

…Continued from previous pages

Author, Year	Sample Description	Sample Size	Research Design	Dosage and Duration	Environmental Intervention Strategies
Lopes *et al.* 2009	International; ELEM; BL BMI in girls 6 – 7 = 16.4; girls 8+ = 17.7; BL BMI in Boys 6 – 7 = 16.8; Boys 8+ = 17.8	*N* = 168; 81 from one school and 87 from another	Quasi-experimental	30 min/day; 2 weeks	Change in physical environment with addition of playground equipment to increase PA during recess
Muckelbauer *et al.* 2009	International; ELEM; Low-income; BL OW Int = 23.4%; Cnt = 25.9%	*N* = 2950; Int = 1641; Cnt = 1309	RCT	Daily (water fountain exposure), four 45-min classroom lessons; 1 year	Installed water fountains, distribute water bottles, classroom lessons
Ploeg *et al.* 2014	International; ELEM; low-income; BL OW/OB Int = 38.3%; Cnt = 31.3%	10 Int schools; 20 Cnt schools	Quasi-experimental	Daily; 2 years	PC; social & physical environmental changes, healthy school policy, playground programs, classroom-based equipment for PA
Sacchetti *et al.* 2013	International; ELEM; BL OW Cnt = 24.1%; Int = 25%; BL OB Cnt = 8.8%; Int = 10.4%	*N* = 428; Int = 212; Cnt = 216	RCT	30 min PA, 2 × 50 min sessions/week of extra PE/week; 2 years	Daily PA program enhanced in duration, intensity, and frequency

Continued on next page…

...Continued from previous pages

Author, Year	Sample Description	Sample Size	Research Design	Dosage and Duration	Environmental Intervention Strategies
Sallis *et al.*	U.S.; MS; Low-income; BL BMI Int boys = 20.1; Int girls = 19.8; Cnt boys = 19.7; Cnt girls =19.5	N = 24 schools with Mean enrollment of 1,109/school	RCT	Daily; 2 years	Change in PE lessons, increased daily PA, modification of school food offerings, implement school nutrition policies
Singh *et al.* 2007	International; MS; Int OW = 9.4%; Int OB = 1.1%; Cnt OW = 16.7%; Cnt OB = 1.3%	N = 1053; Int = 600; Cnt = 453	RCT	8-months; 2 fixed periods throughout the year	Adapted curriculum for 11 biology and PE lessons and additional PE lessons
Wang *et al.* 2010	U.S.; ELEM; Low-income; BL OW/OB not assessed	N = 327; 269 after second year (4 Int groups: 72, 32, 58, 107)	Prospective	Daily; 2 years	PC; Change in school food, school dining, offer cooking classes, school gardens, nutrition lesson integration across academic subjects

Table 1. Summary of included interventions—sample, design, intervention description. BL = Baseline; BMI = Body Mass Index; Cnt = Control Group; ELEM = Elementary; H = Hours; Int = Intervention Group; Min = Minutes; MS = Middle School; OB = Obese; OW = Overweight; PA = Physical Activity; PC = Parental Component; PE = Physical Education; RCT = Randomized Controlled Trial

Author, Year	Primary Outcome(s)	Measures	Measures-Time	Attrition	Salient Findings
Donnelly et al. 2009	BMI	Ht, Wt, academic achievement	BL, 3 years	2.5% dropped out	Change for overweight to at-risk approached sig ($p = 0.08$)
Foster et al. 2008	OW, OB	Ht, Wt questionnaire for dietary intake, PA, sedentary behavior	BL, spring of year 1, 2 years	Int & Cnt schools at 1 (31.9% vs. 31.5%) and 2 years (36.0% vs. 39.2%)	Cnt = 15%, Int = 7.5% OW in 2 years
Graf et al., 2005	BMI and motor abilities (lateral jumping and 6 min run)	Weight, height, BMI, lateral jumping, 6 minute run	BL and 2 years	Not mentioned	Lateral jumps was sig higher in Int ($p < 0.0001$) and for 6 min run, increase in distance run was sig for Int ($p = 0.020$)
Graf et al. 2008	Endurance, motor, coordination tests	Ht, Wt, BMI, motor tests, body coordination tests	BL, year 2, 4	2% dropped out	23.2% of OB and OW children from Int reached normal weight at final exam
Haerens et al., 2006	BMI	Height, weight, BMI	BL, year 1, 2	12.8% did not complete post-measures	In girls, BMI and SMI z-score increased significantly less in the intervention with PC compared with control group ($p < 0.05$) or intervention group alone ($p = 0.05$)

Continued on next page…

...Continued from previous pages

Author, Year	Primary Outcome(s)	Measures	Measures-Time	Attrition	Salient Findings
Hartmann et al. 2010	Physical, psychosocial QOL	QOL (survey), pubertal stages, anthropometry, body composition, sociodemographic variables	BL, 1 year	10% did not have valid post-intervention data	PA had sig effect on psychosocial QOL in OW ($p < 0.05$) and urban first graders ($p < 0.05$)
Hollar et al. 2010	BMI	Ht, Wt, FCAT scores	BL, 2 years	Not mentioned	Decrease BMI between baseline and post-intervention: Cnt OW = 6.8 %, Int = 2.1% ($p = 0.27$)
Johnston et al. 2013	zBMI, academic outcomes	Ht, Wt, GPA	BL, 2 years	21 % did not complete all measures	Students who were OW/OB in the PFI sig reduced (zBMI) compared to SH group ($p < 0.001$)
Lopes et al. 2009	PA levels	Gender, age, BMI. accelerometer	BL, 2-weeks	24 excluded	Sig. effects for total PA ($p < 0.001$). Sig. interaction between gender & age ($p = 0.009$)
Muckelbauer et al. 2009	BMI	Ht, Wt, gender, age, survey	BL, 1 year	8% non-completers	BMI changed from baseline to follow-up 0.005 ± 0.289 in Int & 0.007 ± 0.295 in Cnt
Ploeg et al. 2014	PA	Pedometer, PA log, OB/OW,BMI	BL, 2 years	Attrition at 2 years: Int = 51.9%, Cnt = 54.6%	OW/OB ($p < 0.05$): Int = 35.2% (–3.1% from BL) and Cnt = 30.1% (–1.2% from BL)

Continued on next page...

...Continued from previous pages

Author, Year	Primary Outcome(s)	Measures	Measures-Time	Attrition	Salient Findings
Sacchetti *et al.* 2013	PA, physical performance, BMI	Ht, Wt.t, BMI, motor tests	BL, 2 years	Int = 14.2%, Cnt = 13.9%	Decrease (boys: 10%; girls: 12%) sedentary activities, $p < 0.05$; Int lower rise in BMI compared to Cnt ($p < 0.001$)
Sallis *et al.* 2003	Changes in eating & PA behaviors	Direct observation, surveys	BL, annual, 2 years	40% non-completers at post intervention	Sig intervention effect for PA for total group ($p < 0.009$) and boys ($p < 0.001$), but not girls ($p < 0.40$). Reduced BMI for boys ($p < 0.5$).
Singh *et al.*, 2007	Height & Weight, hip & waist circumference, skinfold thickness, BMI	Waist and hip circumferences, skinfolds, height, weight, BMI	BL, 8 months	7% non completers at post intervention	Sig change hip circumference (mean difference=0.53 cm) and sum of skinfolds among girls (Mean difference, −2.31 mm). In boys, the Int resulted in sig difference in waist circumference (mean difference= -0.57 cm)
Wang *et al.* 2010	Nutrition knowledge, fruits & vegetables	Surveys, food diaries, interviews with teachers & administration			Students most exposed to Int increased fruits & vegetables by 0.2 cups, students least exposed decreased 0.3 cups ($p < 0.05$)

Table 2. Summary of interventions—outcomes, measures, salient findings. BL = Baseline; BMI = Body Mass Index; Cnt = Control Group; Ht = Height; Int = Intervention Group; OB = Obese; OW = Overweight; PA = Physical Activity; QOL = Quality of Life; Sig = Significant; Wt = Weight.

Environmental strategies among the school-based interventions varied, as did the comprehensive nature of a multi-component approach. One third of the interventions focused solely on physical activity environmental changes, four interventions incorporated nutrition environmental changes only, and almost 30% of the interventions included a combination of both nutrition and physical activity environmental changes. The reported strategies are in line with recommendations to enhance obesity prevention efforts in the school setting (DASH *et al.*, 2010; Swinburn *et al.*, 1999; WHO, 2012). These include schools supporting physical activity and healthier food options, promoting high quality health and physical education, setting nutrition standards, and establishing requirements for how much time children need to spend in physical education classes (DASH *et al.*, 2010). Future school-based interventions should integrate a comprehensive environmental approach, to include physical, economic, political, and sociocultural facets (Swinburn *et al.*, 1999). Implementing a Comprehensive School Health Program, similar to Ploeg and colleagues, may be an ideal solution, considering the impact on prevalence of obesity among intervention schools (Ploeg *et al.*, 2014). Complementary strategies might include using state and local data to guide decision-making practices and policies, supporting the development of school health councils, establishing strong wellness policies, and improving school staff with certification and continuing education so that they may be more knowledgeable of practices and better able to provide for students (DASH *et al.*, 2010). The World Health Organization (2012) also encourages supportive environments, policies, and programs which can lead to behavior change and social, environmental, health and economic outcomes. Ideally, future school-based obesity prevention interventions can, and should, build on the aforementioned recommendations to impact the childhood obesity epidemic while considering the feasibility of implementing so many changes at once.

All of the included interventions employed a multi-component approach, with the environmental change(s) highlighted as an integral component of the intervention. Additional intervention strategies were utilized to complement the related environmental strategies and further promote behavior change: physical activity throughout the curriculum, nutrition and/or health education, and staff encouragement to consume healthy food and increase physical activity. Results from this review indicate interventions which integrated both nutrition and physical activity environmental strategies were more likely to result in statistically significant decreases in BMI and/or overweight or obesity. Interventions which integrated health concepts throughout the curriculum found success and maintained very low attrition over duration of 3–4 years (Donnelly *et al.*, 2009; Graf *et al*, 2008). This lends support to a multi-pronged approach which draws upon evidence-based environmental strategies as well as supportive, complementary intervention approaches for increased effectiveness (RWJF, 2013).

Further necessitating the need for school-based obesity prevention interventions emphasizing environmental changes is the undeniable fact that neighborhoods which are socially disadvantaged lack access to outdoor playgrounds and recreational facilities, violence and crime rates make it unsafe for children to play outside, and there is less access to nutritious foods (Davidson *et al.*, 2010; Gidlow & Ellis, 2011; Veugelers *et al.*, 2008). Schools can provide health enhancing environments to which some children would otherwise not be exposed. Given that over half of the schools within this review targeted low-income populations further reinforces the importance and value in implementing school-based prevention interventions. However, future interventions should take into consideration the target population in an effort to ensure strategies are culturally appropriate to increase adherence and retention.

Parental influence with regard to childhood nutrition and physical activity level is known to be a well-documented determinant of childhood obesity (Budd & Hayman, 2006; Rennie *et al.*, 2005; RWJF, 2013; Sharma & Ickes, 2008). In the included interventions, sixty percent mentioned a parental component, with varying degrees of involvement. Five of the seven interventions which targeted low-income schools contained a parental component, of which more than half resulted in significant declines in BMI and/or overweight or obesity (Foster *et al.*, 2008; Hollar *et al.*, 2010; Sallis *et al.*, 2003), lending support to parental involvement as an integral component to successful school-based interventions, particularly in low-income schools. Including a parental component may encourage sustainable behaviors both in and out of school. Although parental involvement was not operationalized specifically as an environmental strategy within this review, future studies might solely consider parental influence as a critical environmental factor and build on the relationship to other environmental strategies (Swinburn *et al.*, 1999). Incorporating evidence-based strategies is vital to the success of school-based obesity prevention interventions. Of equal importance is the use of theory to plan, implement and evaluate said interventions. While research indicates the increased effectiveness of programs which use a theoretical framework as compared to those which do not (Sharma, 2006), only three of the included interventions cited a theoretical framework, the Theory of Planned Behavior. The applicability of the Theory of Planned Behavior in school-based obesity prevention interventions which integrate environmental strategies is difficult to determine based upon the limited evidence resulting from this review. In addition, neither of the two interventions described how the theory was operationalized, making it even more difficult to come to any conclusions. Though the Theory of Planned Behavior is often cited in school-based interventions (Sharma, 2006, 2007), there may be a more appropriate theoretical fit given the importance placed on the environmental changes within the included interventions. Social Cognitive Theory, which has been tested with a number of populations and health behaviors within the school environment (Sharma, 2006), may more fully encompass the comprehensive nature of multi-component school-based interventions. Future research should explore theoretical underpinnings related to school-based obesity prevention efforts.

Over half of the interventions had duration of two or more years, the majority of which resulted in significant BMI reductions. There is a need for school-based interventions of a longer duration, two years or more, particularly when planning and implementing environmental strategies. Most environmental strategies take more time to implement and result in desired outcomes. If the intended outcome is related to obesity indicators such as BMI, it is unlikely that significant results will be apparent immediately following short-term interventions. Consequently, interventions may not be deemed successful, which may or may not be the case. Given that school-based obesity prevention interventions which incorporate environmental strategies have been less studied than other strategies, longitudinal studies would be useful to track changes and allow time for proper implementation.

5   Limitations

Limitations within this review should be noted. As this review was qualitative, data were collected, examined, and summarized in a narrative form; quantitative meta-analysis was not performed. Studies published prior to January 1, 2002 were excluded, though prior systematic reviews were referenced to reinforce the growth of school-based obesity prevention interventions (Sharma, 2006, 2007). Environmental strategies in the area of childhood obesity were not very popular prior to 2002 so this limitation is not likely to greatly affect the results. Environmental strategies are broad in nature (Swinburn et al., 1999) and often included as part of multi-component interventions. Therefore, it was not possible to tease out outcomes solely based on the included environmental strategies. Finally, only peer-reviewed articles within the selected databases were included, which does increase the likelihood of publication bias, as unpublished studies were unreported. Though childhood obesity remains an increasingly popular research topic, the inclusion criteria set forth by the researchers ensured data were collected systematically.

6   Conclusions

The findings of this study reinforce the merit of incorporating environmental changes in school-based childhood obesity prevention interventions (The Community Guide, n.d.). Environmental and policy interventions have been given modest attention in prior research, but studies have indicated their effectiveness (French et al., 2001; Sallis et al., 1995; The Community Guide, n.d.). School-based childhood obesity prevention interventions which include environmental strategies have the ability to significantly affect BMI outcomes. Future research should also investigate the comprehensive nature of school-based environmental strategies, including the physical, economic, political, and sociocultural facets.

References

Budd, G.M., Hayman, L.L. (2006). Childhood obesity: Determinants, prevention and treatment. J Cardiovasc Nurs 2006, 21,437–441.13.

Davidson, Z., Simen-Kapeu, A., Veugelers, P. (2010). Neighborhood determinants of self-efficacy, physical activity, and body weights among Canadian children. Health & Place, 2010, 16,567–572.

Division of Adolescent and School Health, National Center for Chronic Disease Prevention and Health Promotion, Centers for Disease Control and Prevention. (2010). School-Based Obesity Prevention Strategies for State Policymakers 2010, Retrieved from http://stacks.cdc.gov/view/cdc/5799

Donnelly, J. E., Greene, J. L., Gibson, C. A., Smith, B. K., Washburn, R. A., Sullivan, D. K., DuBose, K., Mayo, M. S., Schmelzle, K. H., Ryan, J. J., Jacobsen, D. J., Williams, S. L. (2009). Physical Activity Across the Curriculum (PAAC): a randomized controlled trial to promote physical activity and diminish overweight and obesity in elementary school children. Prev Med 2009, 49, 336–341.

Farris R., Nicklas T., Webber L., Berenson G. (2000). Nutrient contribution of school lunch program: implications for Healthy People 2000. J School Health 1992, 62, 180–184.

Foster, G. D., Sherman, S., Borradaile, K. E., Grundy, K. M., Vander Veur, S. S., Nachmani, J., Karpyn, A., Kumanyika, S.,Shults, J. (2008). A policy-based school intervention to prevent overweight and obesity. Pediatrics 2008, 121, 794–802.

Freedman, D.S., Mei, Z., Srinivasan, S.R., Berenson, G.S., Dietz, W.H.. (2007). Cardiovascular risk factors and excess adiposity among overweight children and adolescents: The bogalusa heart study. J Pediatr 2007, 150, 12–17.

French S.A., Story, M., Perry, C.L. (1995). Self-esteem and obesity in children and adolescents: A literature review. Obes Res 1995, 3, 479–490.

French S., Story M., Jeffery R. (2001). Environmental influences on eating and physical activity. Ann Rev Public Health 2001, 22, 309–335.

Fryar, C.D., Carroll, M.D., Ogden, C.L. (2010). Prevalence of overweight, obesity, and extreme obesity among adults: United States, trends 1960–1962 through 2009–2010. Centers for Disease Control and Prevention 2010. http://www.cdc.gov/nchs/data/hestat/obesity_adult_09_10/obesity_adult_09_10.htm (accessed on 12 May 2014).

Gidlow, C., Ellis, N. (2011). Neighbourhood green space in deprived urban communities: issues and barriers to use. Local Environment, 2011, 16, 989–1002.

Graf, C., Koch, B., Falkowski, G., Jouck, S., Christ, H., Staunmaier, K., Bjarnason-Wehrens, B., Tokarski, W., Dordel, S., Predel, H. (2005). Effects of a school-based intervention on BMI and motor abilities in childhood. J Sport Sci Med 2005, 4, 291–299.

Graf, C., Koch, B., Falkowski, G., Jouck, S., Christ, H., Staudenmaier, K., Tokarski, W., Gerber, A., Predel, H., Dordel, S. (2008). School-based prevention: effects on obesity and physical performance after 4 years. J Sports Sci 2008, 26, 987–994.

Haernes, L., Deforche, B., Maes, L., Stevens, V., Cardon, G., De Bourdeaudhuij, I. (2006). Body mass effects of a physical activity and healthy food intervention in middle schools. Obesity 2006, 14, 847–854.

Hartmann, T., Zahner, L., Pühse, U., Puder, J. J., Kriemler, S. (2010). Effects of a school-based physical activity program on physical and psychosocial quality of life in elementary school children: a cluster-randomized trial. Pediatric   Exercise Science 2010, 22, 511–522.

Hollar, D., Messiah, S.E., Lopez-Mitnik, G., Hollar, T.L., Almon, M., Agatston, A.S. (2010). Effect of a two-year obesity prevention intervention on percentile changes in body mass index and academic performance in low-income elementary school children. Am J Public Health 2010, 100, 646–653.

Johnston, C.A., Moreno, J.P., El-Mubasher, A., Gallagher, M., Tyler, C., Woehler, D.(2013). Impact of a School-Based Pediatric Obesity Prevention Program Facilitated by Health Professionals. J Sch Health 2013, 83, 171–181.

Lopes, L., Lopes, V., Pereira, B. (2009). Physical activity levels in normal weight and overweight Portuguese children: an intervention study during an elementary school recess. International Electronic Journal of Health Education 2009, 12, 175–184.

Muckelbauer, R., Libuda, L., Clausen, K., Toschke, A. M., Reinehr, T., Kersting, M. (2009). Promotion and provision of drinking water in schools for overweight prevention: randomized, controlled cluster trial. Pediatrics 2009, 123, 661–667.

Myers L., Strikmiller P., Webber L,, Berenson G. (1996). Physical and sedentary activity in school children grades 5–8: the Bogalusa Heart Study. Med Sci Sports Exerc 1996, 28, 852–859.

Ogden, C.L., Carroll, M.D., Kit, B.K., Flegal, K.M. (2012). Prevalence of obesity and trends in body mass index among US children and adolescents, 1999–2010. JAMA 2012, 307, 483–490.

Olds, T., Maher, C., Zumin, S., Peneau, S., Lioret, S., Castetbon, K., Bellisle, De Wilde, J., Hohepa, M., Maddison, R., Lissner, L., Sjoberg, A., Zimmermann, M., Aeberli, I., Ogden, C., Flegal, K., Summerbell C. (2011). Evidence that the prevalence of childhood overweight is plateauing: data from nine countries. International Journal of Pediatric Obesity 2011, 6, 342–260.

Onis, M., Blossner, M., Borghi, E. (2010). Global prevalence and trends of overweight and obesity among preschool children. Am J Clin Nutr 2010, 92, 1257–1264.

Ploeg, K., Maximova, K., McGavock, J., Davis, W., Veugelers, P. (2014). Do school-based physical activity interventions increase or reduce inequalities in health? Soc Sci Med 2014, 112, 80– 87.

Rennie, K.L., Johnson, L., Jebb, S.A. (2005). Behavioural determinants of obesity. Best Prac Res Clin Anaesthesiol 2005, 19, 343–358. 112.

Robert Wood Johnson Foundation. (2013). F as in fat: How obesity threatens America's future. RWJF 2013, Washington, DC.

Ross J., Gilbert G. (1985). The National Children and Youth Fitness Study: A summary of findings. J Physical Educ Recreat Dance 1985, 56, 45–50.

Sacchetti, R., Ceciliani, A., Garulli, A., Dallolio, L.' Beltrami, P., Leoni, E. (2013). Effects of a 2-Year School-Based Intervention of Enhanced Physical Education in the Primary School. J Sch Health 2013, 83, 639–646.

Sallis J., Chen A., Castro C. (1995). School-based interventions for childhood obesity. In: Cheung

L., Richmond J., eds. *Child health, nutrition, and physical activity. Champaign, IL: Human Kinetics 1995; 179–204.*

Sallis, J., McKenzie, T., Conway, T., Elder, J., Prochaska, J., Brown, M., Zive, M., Marshall, S., Alcarez, J. (2003). *Environmental interventions for eating and physical activity: a randomized controlled trial in middle schools. Am J Prev Med 2003, 24, 209–217.*

Sharma, M. (2006). *School-based interventions for childhood and adolescent obesity. Obes Rev 2006, 7, 261–269.*

Sharma, M. (2007). *International school-based interventions for preventing obesity in children. Obes Rev 2007, 8, 155–167.*

Sharma, M., Ickes, J. (2008). *Psychological determinants of childhood and adolescent obesity. JSBHS 2008, 2, 33–49.*

Singh, A., Paw, M., Brug, J., van Mechelen, W. (2007). *Short term effects of school-based weight gain prevention among adolescents. Arch Pediatr Adolesc Med 2007, 161, 565–571.*

Summerbell C.D., Edmunds, L. D., Kelly, S., Brown, T., Campbell, K. J. (2005). *Interventions for preventing obesity in children. Cochrane Systematic Review 2005, 3.*

Swinburn, B., Egger, G., Raza, F. (1999). *Dissecting obesogenic environments: The development and application of a framework for identifying and prioritizing environmental interventions for obesity. Prev Med 1999, 29, 563–570.*

The Community Guide. *Obesity prevention and control: School-based programs. http://www. thecommunityguide.org/obesity/schoolbased.html (accessed on 18 January 2014).*

Veugelers, P., Sithole, F., Zhang, S., Muhajarine, N. (2008). *Neighborhood characteristics in relation to diet, physical activity, and overweight of Canadian children.* Int J Pediatr Obes *2008, 3, 152–159.*

Wang, M.C., Rauzon, S., Studer, N., Martin, A.C., Craig, L., Merlo, C., Kursunoglu, D., Shannguan, M., Crawford, P. (2010). *Exposure to a comprehensive school intervention increases vegetable consumption. J Adolesc Health 2010, 47, 74–82.*

Whitlock E.P., Williams S.B., Gold R., Smith P.R., Shipman S.A.(2005). *Screening and interventions for childhood overweight: A summary of evidence for the US Preventive Services Task Force. Pediatrics 2005, 116, 125–144.*

Withrow, D., Alter, D.A. (2011). *The economic burden of obesity worldwide: A systematic review of the direct costs of obesity. Obesity Rev 2011, 12, 131–141.*

World Health Organization. (2012). *Population based approaches to childhood obesity prevention. 2012, Retrieved from http://www.who.int/dietphysicalactivity/childhood/ approaches/en/*

Young, B.E, Johnson, S.L., Krebs, N.F. (2012). *Advances in nutrition. Adv Nutr 2012, 3, 675–686.*

Chapter 3

Cost Effectiveness of Bariatric Surgery as a Treatment for Morbid Obesity: A Literature Review

Muhammad Ali Karim[1], Sumiya Altaf[2], W Gordon Mackay[3] and AbdulMajid Ali[4]

1   Background

Obesity is no less than an epidemic with current reports forecasting a substantial strain on health economies if appropriate intervention is not actively instituted. It is estimated that there are 1.1 billion adults worldwide that are classified as being overweight or obese (Haslam & James, 2005). The rising prevalence of obesity is a major public health concern as excess body weight has significant health implications, in particular cardiovascular disease, diabetes mellitus, musculoskeletal problems and cancer (Clinical Guidelines on the Identification, 1998).

According to the Public Health England report 2014, 24.7% of adults aged 16 years and above are obese (body mass index $\geq 30\text{kg/m}^2$) and the prevalence of obesity in England has significantly increased since 1993 (National Obesity Observatory, 2014). By 2015, the Foresight Report estimates that 36% of males and 28% of females aged between 21 and 60 years of age will become obese. By 2050, it is predicted that obesity will affect up to 60% of adult men, 50% of adult women and 25% of children (Butland *et al.*, 2007).

[1] Department of Surgery, University Hospital Ayr, UK

[2] King AbdulAziz Medical City, UK

[3] Institute of Healthcare Associated Infection, University of the West of Scotland, UK

[4] Consultant General and Upper GI Surgeon, University Hospital Ayr, University of the West of Scotland, UK

At present, obesity costs the UK economy £7 billion and the National Health Service (NHS) £2 billion per year. The projected future costs to the economy may increase to a staggering £45 billion with costs to the NHS £6.5 billion by the year 2050 (Butland *et al.*, 2007).

The escalation of obesity has resulted in bariatric surgery becoming more readily available and gaining popularity. The estimated number of bariatric operations performed in the United States alone in 2008 was thirteen-fold higher than the number performed in 1992 (Dumon & Murayam, 2011).

Types of bariatric operations may be classified as either restrictive, malabsorptive or a combination of both. Restrictive procedures include adjustable gastric band (AGB), vertical banded gastroplasty (VGB), sleeve gastrectomy and intragastric balloon insertion (Elder & Wolfe, 2007; Stanczyk *et al.*, 2007). Malabsorptive procedures include biliopancreatic diversion/ duodenal switch and jejunoileal bypass (Shabbir *et al.*, 2009). Roux-en-Y gastric bypass (RYGB) is a commonly performed procedure that is both restrictive and malabsorptive (Maggard *et al.*, 2005). Since the advent of laparoscopic approach and further development of techniques in bariatric surgery, there has been a reduction in post-operative complications and overall improved favourable outcomes after surgery (Abell & Minocha, 2006; Hutter *et al.*, 2006; Reoch *et al.*, 2011).

There is ongoing research investigating the outcomes of bariatric surgery, both at regional and national levels. There are already several published studies that explore the health benefits of bariatric surgery with focus on patients' quality of life and obesity-related health conditions (Ashrafian *et al.*, 2008; Buchwald *et al.*, 2004; Sjöström *et al.*, 2004; 2012).

Cost saving is a term applicable to preventative care that decreases future costs. When the outcomes of an intervention are significant then this is considered to be cost effective (Goodell *et al.*, 2009).

A number of published economic evaluation studies have demonstrated the impact of bariatric surgery on health services and economics. With the advent of weight loss surgery being relatively new, long term outcomes remain largely unclear. The purpose of this review is to address the early cost effectiveness of bariatric surgery and speculate on long term health and financial benefits.

2   Search Structure and Methodology

2.1   Data Sources and Study Selection

A comprehensive electronic search of Ovid database was performed. Ovid, MEDLINE, EMBASE, EBM Reviews: Cochrane Database of Systematic Reviews and EBM Reviews: Cochrane Central Register of Clinical Trials, NHS Economic Evaluations Database and Health Technology Assessments Database were searched for all relevant articles written in the English language that described cost effectiveness of bariatric procedures in adult populations (age > 18 years). All clinical trials and economic evaluation studies published from 1996–2012 were searched for relevant articles.

Data was searched for articles comparing either:

- Cost effectiveness of bariatric surgery versus medical treatment (diet and exercise) / pharmacological treatments) for obesity

- Pre- and post-operative cost implications of different bariatric procedures

- Direct and indirect economic impact of bariatric surgery on health care systems

- Impact of bariatric surgery on quality of life, morbidity related to obesity, cost effectiveness in QALY

Full articles were retrieved applying the selection criteria to the abstracts and titles. Randomised controlled trials (RCT), perspective cohort studies, retrospective cohort studies and articles describing laparoscopic or open bariatric procedures were included. All included articles were obtained and read by two reviewers. The findings were discussed and tabulated (see Table 1). Literature reviews and studies on animals, childhood obesity or those without clear outcomes on the cost effectiveness of bariatric surgery and any publication not in the English language were excluded.

2.2 Primary Economic Evaluation

In this review, all three types of economic evaluations were included (cost benefit analysis, cost effectiveness analysis and cost utility analysis) in order to obtain a detailed representation of economic evaluations carried out in the field of bariatric surgery. The direct impact on health care services can be measured by assessing the outcomes of bariatric surgery patients compared to non-surgical groups in terms of excess weight loss, gained QALY, improved or resolved comorbid conditions like diabetes, reduction in medications, decreased hospital visits or in-hospital stays and incremental cost and cost effectiveness ratios (ICER). Below the terms used in economic evaluation s are briefly explained

Cost benefit analysis: Cost benefit analysis shows the overall costs and benefits of an intervention. It evaluates the excess of monetary benefits over the costs (Palmer *et al.*, 1999).

Cost utility analysis: Cost utility analysis measures the effect of an intervention on both the quantitative and qualitative aspects of health using measures such as Quality Adjusted Life Years (QALY's) gained (Waxman, 2013).

Cost effectiveness analysis (CEA): Cost effectiveness analysis shows what it costs to achieve a certain effect. In cost effectiveness analysis, costs and benefits are measured in non-comparable units e.g., life years gained, improvement in physical health status etc.

The incremental cost-effectiveness ratio (ICER): ICER of an intervention is defined "as the ratio of the change in costs of a therapeutic intervention (compared to the alternative, such as doing nothing or using the best available alternative treatment) to the change in effects of the intervention" (Waxman, 2013).

Direct costs of obesity consist of expenditure on disease prevention, diagnosis and treatment. Indirect costs of obesity include reduced economic output mortality, decreased productivity at work, unemployment and decreased time at work.

2.3   Methodology of Cost Effectiveness Studies

The economic evaluation studies included in our research are RCTs, observational case control studies and prospective studies based on an economic model or a decision tree. Cost effectiveness analysis of bariatric surgery is usually performed using decision trees or Markov models to estimate the effects prospectively over a long time frame. For this review, data was extracted from previously published studies, health databases and payer-sourced cost data. This selection also comprises of sensitivity testing used for each model. This can aid policy makers and health economists to evaluate the benefits of bariatric services provision in a given population.

3   Search Results

A total of 949 articles were obtained at the first stage of the search. Seventy five articles met the inclusion criteria in the second stage. Further exclusion resulted in 36 articles in the third stage. Full articles were then extracted and a fourth stage manual search was carried out that yielded 26 relevant articles with clear methodology and outcomes.

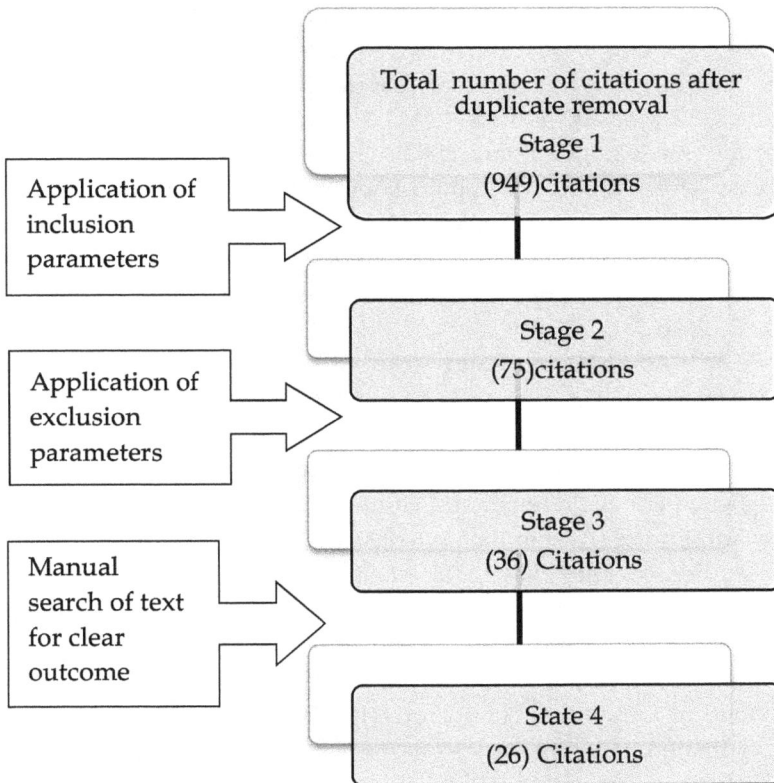

Figure 1 Flow chart of search methodology and structure.

4   Descriptive and Tabular Analysis of Relevant Studies

At the end of the structured search strategy, 26 relevant articles were to be included in this literature review. There were seven RCTs, ten model-based observational studies, six retrospective cohort studies and three case-control observational studies. To achieve comprehensive and organized data results, these 26 studies are categorised by their primary objectives.

4.1   Bariatric surgery versus No Treatment/Standard Treatment

This group included studies comparing costs of either bariatric surgery versus no treatment for obese patients, bariatric surgery versus standard medical treatment for obese patients or specific bariatric procedure versus no treatment or standard care.

In this group were 16 articles. A comprehensive description of methodology, results and conclusions of these studies is shown in Table 1. Of all studies comparing bariatric surgery with no treatment or standard care, 11 studies reported cost effectiveness results of bariatric surgery as costs / QALYs gained. Five studies have estimated direct economic impact of bariatric procedures on health services. From the payers' perspective, the long term cost utility of surgery compared to non-surgical management is convincing with ICUR ranging from $1,000–$40,000 per QALY.

A study by Craig et al. estimated cost effectiveness of gastric bypass surgery compared to no treatment and reported that gastric bypass surgery is dominantly cost effective with ICER = $5,000–$16,100 / QALY for women and $10,000–$35,600 / QALY for men over lifetime (Craig & Tseng, 2002).

The cost effectiveness of laparoscopic adjustable gastric band (AGB) and laparoscopic Roux-en-Y gastric bypass (RYGB) as treatment for morbid obesity was compared to no treatment. This study by Campbell et al. showed 100% probability that AGB and RYGB are cost effective over lifetime at willingness to pay of $50,000 (Campbell et al., 2010).

Studies by Anselmino et al and Ackroyd et al. were based on health economic models and compared cost effectiveness of bariatric surgery to the standard care treatment of obese patients in six European countries. The results showed that both adjustable gastric band and Roux-en-Y gastric bypass are cost effective over a period of 5 years in diabetic patients in Spain and United Kingdom, and cost saving in Germany, Austria, Italy and France (Anselmino et al., 2009; Ackroyd et al., 2006).

Three studies (Makary et al., 2010; Maciejewski et al., 2010; Crémieux et al., 2008) have estimated the overall pre-operative, operative and post-operative economic impact of bariatric surgery. They have shown similar results with immediate post-operative costs being higher as compared to the pre-operative period but these costs adopt a downward trend at 6 months post-operatively. Fifteen months after surgery, monthly savings are estimated to be around $400–$600 for open bariatric procedures ($p < 0.01$) and > $900 for laparoscopic bariatric surgery in as early as 13 months following surgery ($p < 0.01$). This decline in the cost post-operatively is attributed to the decrease in medication use, number of outpatient clinics and laboratory investigations especially in

Reference	Efficacy Data (study design, methods, model)	Aim of Study	Population (BMI, age, DM)	Comparators	Base Case (incremental cost, QALY), Time horizon	Sensitivity Analysis
Makary *et al.*, 2010	Retrospective time series; 2,235 obese type 2 DM patients 2002 – 2005	To study medication utilisation and annual health care costs in patients with type 2 DM before and after bariatric surgery	Mean age 48.4 years, type 2 DM	Bariatric surgery (pre- and post-op), pharmacological treatment	Pre-procedure health care cost = $6376 Mean procedure cost = $29,959 Post-procedure cost: Year 1 = 10% more than pre-op Year 2 = 34% less Year 3 = 70% less	After surgery, the proportion using at least one diabetic medication decreased to 25.3% at 6 months, 19.4% at 12 months, and 15.5% at 24 months
Hoerger *et al.*, 2010	CDC-RTI (Centre for Disease Control and Prevention - RTI Diabetes cost effectiveness model)	Cost effectiveness of bariatric surgery in patients with type 2 DM (newly diagnosed and obese patients with established DM)	BMI ≥ 30, age 35-74 years, DM	AGB, RYGB, standard care	*RYGB* = $7000/QALY, 2.21 QALYs gained (incident DM); $12,000/QALY, 1.70 QALY's gained (prevalent DM) *AGB* = $11,000/QALY, 1.57 QALYs gained (incident DM); $13,000/QALY, 1.34 QALYs gained (prevalent DM)	95% probability that RYGB cost effective for 45 – 54 years ranged from $2,300 – $27,000; 95% probability that AGB cost effective for 45 – 54 years ranged from $0 – $35,000

Continued on next page...

. . . Continued from previous pages

Keating *et al.*, 2009	2 year randomized control trial, 60 obese patients in Australia	To determine the within trial cost efficacy of surgical therapy relative to conventional therapy for achieving remission of DM in class I and II obese patients	BMI 30 – 40, recently diagnosed type 2 DM	Laparoscopic AGB, standard care	ICER for conventional therapy compared to no intervention = 25,500AUD/DM remission case; ICER for surgical compared to conventional therapy = 16,600AUD/DM remission case; Time horizon = 2 years	Mean duration of DM remission must be ≥ 2 years to be cost effective, ≥ 10 years to be dominant
Maciejewski *et al.*, 2010	Retrospective longitudinal cohort study of health care use and expenditures from 2000 – 2006; 846 obese veteran patients	To examine health care utilization and expenditures of severely obese individuals before and after bariatric surgery within the veterans health administration	Mean BMI = 48.5, mean age 51 years, 73% males	Bariatric surgery pre-op expenditure versus post-op expenditure	Expenditures increased nearly $549 ($p < 0.001$) every 6 months of the pre-surgical period and decreased $346 ($p < 0.001$) every 6 months of the post-surgical period; Time horizon = 3 years before and after surgery	Adjusted total outpatient, inpatient and overall expenditures all lower in the post-surgical period (all, $p < 0.0001$) post-surgical outpatient medication fills and outpatient laboratory expenditures higher in post-surgical period ($p < 0.0001$)

Continued on next page...

...Continued from previous pages

Study	Design	Aim	Population	Intervention	Outcomes	Conclusions
Keating et al., 2009	Randomized control trial, 60 obese patients in Australia	To determine the within trial cost efficacy of surgical therapy relative to conventional therapy for achieving DM remission in class I and II obese patients (modeled life time analysis)	BMI 30 – 40, recently diagnosed type 2 DM	Laparoscopic AGB, standard care	Health care savings = 2,400AUD QALYs gained = 1.2/patient Time horizon = life time	Probability of surgical therapy being dominant is 57% with DM remission in ≥ 2 years and for being cost effective is 98% with DM remission in ≥ 10 years
Crémieux et al., 2008	Case control observational study, 3651 cases and 3651 controls, multivariate study 1999 – 2005	A study on the economic impact of bariatric surgery	BMI ≥ 40, mean age = 44 years, 86% females, 10 common comorbid conditions in both groups	Bariatric surgery; standard care	15 months after surgery monthly savings > $500 for the whole sample, $400 – $600 for open bariatric procedure (p < 0.01), laparoscopic bariatric surgery > $900 at 13 months following surgery (p < 0.01)	Costs associated with open surgery are recovered within 49 months (95% CI, 35 – 63 months) Costs associated with laparoscopic surgery are recovered within 25 months (95% CI, 16 – 34 months)

Continued on next page...

...Continued from previous pages

Study	Design / Population	Objective	Population characteristics	Comparators	Cost / outcomes	Results
McEwen et al., 2010	Randomized control trial, 221 patients 2001 - 2005	To assess cost, quality of life impact and the cost utility of bariatric surgery	Mean BMI = 52, mean age = 42 years, 88% females, 36% DM, managed care population	97% RYGB; standard care	Incremental cost/QALY = $48,662 (2 years), $1,425 (lifetime)	$11,345 (lifetime) in non-DM vs. $8,831 in DM, $1,246 for laparoscopic RYGB vs. $17,372 for open RYGB
Maklin et al., 2011	Prospective study based on Markov model and decision tree	To evaluate the cost-utility of bariatric surgery compared to ordinary treatment in Finnish health care system	Mean BMI = 47, mean age = 43 years, 35% males, DM	AGB, RYGB, SG, standard care	Incremental cost of bariatric vs. standard care = -23,375€, AGB = -7,476€, RYGB = -17,288€, SG = -15,733€ Time horizon = 10 years	All bariatric procedures show strong dominance over standard care (1.5x more expensive over 10 years)
Hayashi et al., 2011	Retrospective cohort study, n = 176, 94 bariatric population (group I), 34 clinical (group II), 48 surgical controls (group III)	Four year hospital resource utilization after bariatric surgery: comparison with clinical and surgical controls	Group I BMI = 52.2 ± 10; Group II BMI = 33.8 ± 5; Group III BMI = 23.8 ± 4; age = 18 - 59 years, all females, DM	RYGB; standard care, colorectal surgery	Outpatient visits: Group I = 5.7 ± 0.2/year, Group II = 10.5 ± 0.9/year, Group III = 3.5 ± 0.8/year Time horizon = 5 years	RYGB patients needed 45.8% less outpatient visits and 53% less laboratory tests than other groups

Continued on next page...

...Continued from previous pages

Salem et al., 2008	Based on payer-perspective decision analytic model of 3 year operative and non-operative interventions for morbid obesity	To evaluate the incremental cost effectiveness of bariatric procedures compared with non-operative weight loss interventions and with each other	BMI = 40 – 60, Age = 35 – 55 years, 0% DM	Laparoscopic AGB, laparoscopic RYGB, standard care	ICER in males = $11,604/QALY for AGB compared with $18,543/QALY for RYGB; ICER in females = $8878/QALY for AGB compared with $14,680/QALY for RYGB (lifetime)	Both operations were cost effective at < $25,000/QALY
Sampalis et al., 2004	Observational two cohort study between 1986 – 2002, bariatric group n = 1,035, control group n = 5,746	To assess the impact of weight reduction surgery on health related costs	BMI = 38 – 69, mean age = 45 years, 0% DM	RYGB, VBG, standard care	5 years absolute difference of cumulative costs = CDN $6,000,000 per 1,000 patients in both groups	Initial costs of surgery can be amortized over 3.5 years; RYGB alone reduces 29% of total direct health care costs
Craig et al., 2002	Observational study, n = 608 14 years	To estimate the cost effectiveness of RYGB in the treatment of severe obesity	BMI = 40 – 50, age = 35 – 55 years, 0% DM	RYGB, no treatment	ICER = $5000 – $16,100/QALY for women, $10,000 – $35,600/QALY for men (lifetime)	RYGB is cost effective sensitive to excess weight loss

Continued on next page....

...Continued from previous pages

Ikramuddin *et al.*, 2009	Prospective observational study based on CORE diabetes model, *n* = 204, 2 years	To assess the cost effectiveness of RYGB compared to medical management for treating type 2 DM	Mean BMI = 48.4, mean age = 50 years, 78% females, 100% DM	RYGB; standard care	ICER = $23,510/QALY gained Time horizon = 35 years	84% probability that RYGB cost effective over 35 years at a willingness to pay of $50,000
Anselmino *et al.*, 2009	Perspective observational study based on health economics model in Austria, Italy and Spain	To assess cost effectiveness and budget impact of obesity surgery in type 2 DM in three European countries	BMI ≥35, 100% DM	AGB, RYGB, standard care	*Austria* AGB = −2861€/QALY RYGB = −1447€/QALY *Italy* AGB = −1077€/QALY RYGB = −1246€/QALY *Spain* AGB = 1456€/QALY RYGB = 2664€/QALY (5 years)	AGB and RYGB are cost effective over 5 years time in DM patients in Spain and are cost saving in Austria and Italy

Continued on next page...

...Continued from previous pages

Ackroyd et al., 2006	Perspective observational study based on health economics model in Germany, UK and France	To assess cost effectiveness and budget impact of obesity surgery in type 2 DM in three European countries	BMI ≥ 35, 100% DM	AGB, RYGB, standard care	*Germany* AGB = -3488€/QALY RYGB = -3754€/QALY *France* AGB = -4357€/QALY RYGB = -4385€/QALY *UK* AGB = 1929£/QALY RYGB = 1517£/QALY Time horizon = 5 years	AGB and RYGB are effective at 5 year follow up and cost saving in Germany and France; cost effective in the UK
Campbell et al., 2010	RCT, n = 43 5 years	To assess cost effectiveness of laparoscopic AGB and RYGB as treatment for morbid obesity	BMI > 35, mean age = 40 years, 82% females, 2% DM	Laparoscopic AGB; laparoscopic RYGB; no treatment	Incremental costs/QALY gained $6,033 (lifetime) $6,256 (lifetime)	100% probability that laparoscopic AGB and RYGB are cost effective over lifetime at willingness to pay of $50,000

Table 1: Cost Effectiveness of Bariatric Surgery compared to No Treatment / Non-Surgical Treatment of Obesity. Abbreviations: AGB, adjustable gastric band; AUD, Australian dollar; BMI, body mass index; DM, diabetes mellitus; QALY, quality adjusted life year; RCT, randomised controlled trial; RYGB, Roux-en-Y gastric bypass; SG, sleeve gastrectomy; VBG, vertical banded gastroplasty

diabetic patients (Hayashi *et al.*, 2011). Conclusively according to these studies, the overall cost of the procedure performed is recuperated by the third post-operative year.

An economic evaluation by Sampalis *et al.* showed the initial costs of surgery can be amortised over 3.5 years (Sampalis *et al.*, 2004). It also showed that gastric bypass surgery alone reduces 29% of the total direct health care costs. Cost effectiveness analysis of studies shows that bariatric procedures are most effective clinically and economically in diabetic obese patients compared to non-surgical treatment. The outcomes of four studies (Makary *et al.*, 2010; Hoerger *et al.*, 2010; Keating *et al.*, 2009; Keating *et al.*, 2009) have all shown improvement or remission of diabetes mellitus after surgery with a significant decrease of up to 70% in diabetic medications by these patients in the third post-operative year and ICURs of $7,000–$10,000 over a 10 year time horizon. Mean duration of diabetes remission must be > 2 years to be cost effective and > 10 years to be cost saving.

According to Maklin *et al.* all types of bariatric procedures show strong dominance over conventional care which is 1.5 times more expensive over a 10 year period (Maklin *et al.*, 2011). A previous study Salem *et al.* concluded that both laparoscopic RYGB and laparoscopic AGB were cost effective at $25,000 / QALY (Salem *et al.*, 2008). Among different types of commonly performed bariatric procedures, AGB has led to an increased QALY gained and cost savings when compared to non-surgical management in the diabetic population (Maklin *et al.*, 2011).

4.2 Comparison of Different Bariatric Procedures

This group includes studies comparing costs of either:

* One type of bariatric surgery to another
* Laparoscopic bariatric procedures versus open bariatric procedures
* Longitudinal cost-benefit analysis of one type of bariatric surgery
* Direct and indirect economic impacts of one type of bariatric surgery

A total of eight studies were included in this group. Two of the studies compared the cost of selected procedures, two studies mentioned direct and indirect cost effects of a single procedure and other studies showed the longitudinal cost analysis (cost-benefit analysis) of a single procedure. A comprehensive tabular description of these studies along with their methodology, search results and conclusions is shown in Table 2.

Three, studies have compared the costs of laparoscopic RYGB, laparoscopic AGB and laparoscopic VBG (Nguyen *et al.*, 2001; 2009; Ojo & Valin, 2009). Their results conclude that RYGB is the most costly procedure, followed by AGB and VBG. These costs are incurred as RYGB is a lengthier and technically complex operation requiring further equipment for multiple anastomoses. AGB and VBG have comparable pre-operative and immediate post-operative costs but the intra-operative cost of instruments is greater for AGB.

Laparoscopic procedures are more cost effective when compared to open bariatric procedures despite their higher initial cost of surgery which is adequately offset by lower inpatient hospital costs, shorter hospital stay and post-surgical outcomes in terms of weight loss, less post-operative complications and improved quality of life (Crémieux *et al.*, 2009; McEwen *et al.*, 2010; Nguyen *et al.*, 2001).

Reference	Efficacy Data (study design, methods, model)	Aim of Study	Population (BMI, age, DM)	Comparators	Base Case (incremental cost, QALY, Time horizon)	Sensitivity Analysis
Nguyen et al., 2009	Prospective randomized trial, $n = 250$ 2002 – 2007	To compare the outcomes, quality of life, and costs of laparoscopic RYGB vs. laparoscopic AGB	BMI = 35 – 60, age = 18 – 60 years, 0% DM	Laparoscop-ic RYGB, laparoscopic AGB	Total costs: RYGB = $12,310 AGB = $10,766 ($p < 0.01$)	RYGB costs more than AGB due to longer operative time and hospitalisation
Finkelstein et al., 2011	Cost benefit analysis based on medical claims data 2006 – 2008 MEPS $n = 134$ NHWS $n = 2164$	To estimate direct and indirect costs and potential savings of laparoscopic AGB among obese DM patients	BMI ≥ 35, age = 18 – 64 years, 20% DM	Laparoscop-ic AGB	Net savings in 5 years increase from $26,000 to $34,000 when indirect costs are included	Inclusion of indirect costs improves the financial outlook for laparoscopic AGB
Ojo et al., 2008	Prospective non-randomised study, laparoscopic VBG $n = 59$, laparoscopic AGB $n = 83$ 2005 – 2006	To compare the cost of two gastric restrictive procedures	BMI = meeting criteria for surgery, age = 18 – 65 years	Laparoscop-ic VBG, laparoscopic AGB	Pre-op and immediate post-op cost similar in both; laparoscopic AGB instruments cost, band fills costs and post-op complications are higher	VBG required less expensive instruments and materials and was associated with a higher rate of weight loss and fewer complications

Continued on next page…

...Continued from previous pages

Gemert *et al.*, 1999	Prospective study, *n* = 21	To estimate the direct and indirect cost effectiveness of VBG for the treatment of morbid obesity	Mean BMI = 47.2, mean age = 33.1 years, 24% DM	VBG	VBG total costs = $5,865; QALY gained after VBG = 12 years; increase in paid labour from 19%–48%	For treatment of morbid obesity VBG saves $4,004 – $3,928/QALY
Nguyen *et al.*, 2006	Retrospective study, *n* = 77	To estimate the reduction in prescription medication costs after laparoscopic RYGB	BMI = 38 – 65, age = 17 – 63 years, 71% females, 34% DM	Laparoscop-ic RYGB	Significant reduction in medication use after surgery, medication discontinue rate was 98% GERD, 87% HTN, 85% DM, 87% hyperlipidemia	Mean cost saving per patient after 1 year post- op $168/month, $2016/year
Finkelstein *et al.*, 2011	Retrospective case control study, cases *n* = 7310, controls *n* = 7306	To quantify the costs and potential cost savings resulting from coverage for laparoscopic AGB using a claims analysis	BMI > 35, mean age = 44 years, 12% DM	Laparoscop-ic AGB	Net cost of coverage for laparoscopic AGB was reduced to 0 by approx 4 years after band placement in non-DM and 2 years in DM patients	Laparoscopic AGB procedure pays for itself within a relatively short period, especially for those with DM

Continued on next page...

…Continued from previous pages

Mullen *et al.*, 2010	Observational pre–post test design, *n* = 224 2000-2007	To assess the effect of RYGB surgery on the total cost of medical care for morbidly obese members	BMI ≥ 30, mean age = 43 years, 82% females	RYGB	Surgical costs recouped at 3.5 years post-surgery	Longitudinal costs savings for patients undergoing RYGB surgery are cost effective
Nguyen *et al.*, 2001	Prospective randomised trial, laparoscopic RYGB *n* = 79, open RYGB *n* = 76, 1999-2001	To compare outcomes, quality of life and costs of laparoscopic and open RYGB	BMI = 40 – 60, mean age = 40 years	Laparoscopi-c RYGB, open RYGB	Operative costs are higher for laparoscopic RYGB but hospital costs are lower	Laparoscopic RYGB is safe and cost effective alternative to open RYGB for morbid obesity

Table 2: Comparison of Cost Effectiveness / Longitudinal Cost Analysis of different Bariatric Procedures. Abbreviations: AGB, adjustable gastric band; BMI, body mass index; DM, diabetes mellitus; GERD, gastroesophageal reflux disease; HTN, hypertension; MEPS, Medical Expenditure Panel Survey; NHWS, National Health and Wellness Survey; QALY, quality adjusted life year; RYGB, Roux-en-Y gastric bypass; VBG, vertical banded gastroplasty

Net cost savings per QALY of three commonly performed bariatric procedures are as follows:

- Vertical banded gastroplasty = $4,004–$3,928 / QALY (Nguyen *et al.*, 2006)

- Roux-en-Y gastric bypass = $23,000 / QALY (Ikramuddin *et al.*, 2009)

- Adjustable gastric band = $25,000 / QALY (Salem *et al.*, 2008)

4.3   Studies Showing the Effect of Bariatric Surgery on Paid Employment

Two studies were included which addressed the subsequent indirect effect, with focus on employment potential. A case series survey undertaken in southwest England by *Hawkins et al.* in which 59 patients were assessed for a mean of 14 months after bariatric surgery. The proportion in paid work rose from 58% before surgery, to 76% after surgery which was comparable to the normal population average. There was also 57% increase in total time worked per week. The total number of benefits claimed had fallen by 75% (Hawkins *et al.*, 2007).

Ewing *et al.* carried out a cost-benefit analysis of bariatric surgery in the southern plains of Texas from 2003–2005. Their findings showed obesity led to a loss of 1,977 jobs and decreased indirect business tax revenues by over $13 million per year. Bariatric surgery yields an economic benefit of between $1.3–$9.9 billion. The net benefit consists of the upfront costs of the surgical procedure and ongoing gains from improvements in each individual's productivity (Ewing *et al.*, 2001).

5   Limitations and Potential for Future Studies

Most of the studies included in our review are prospective observational studies based on economic models. The major limitation of published cost effectiveness models is that observational data and relatively short term RCT data were used to model the long term impacts. These models may overestimate the economic attractiveness of weight loss surgery despite carrying out a wide range of sensitivity analysis. Further models will be more relevant if they include population-based estimates of risk and outcomes and more accurate payer-sourced cost data.

There is a lack of long term RCTs comparing the outcomes and economic impact of each bariatric procedure. This is required in order to conclude the most appropriate and cost effective surgical procedure recommended for a defined group of obese individuals.

Most of the studies measure the cost effectiveness of surgery by calculating the direct immediate costs on health care resources. Although this is easily calculated, it is however incomplete as it does not account for post-operative indirect costs. Further studies that incorporate indirect costs would provide a more comprehensive sum of the economic impact of bariatric surgery.

Exclusion of non-English language studies and studies that did not show cost effectiveness of bariatric surgery and were not published may also be a source of bias.

6   Conclusion

Based upon published literature, bariatric surgery is cost effective in short term analysis and cost saving over a prolonged period of time compared to conventional treatment for obesity. The comparison between all types of bariatric procedures shows strong dominance over traditional care which is 1.5 times more costly over 10 years.

Both open and laparoscopic bariatric surgery is cost effective. However laparoscopic surgery appears more cost effective when compared with open surgery. Costs associated with open surgery can be recovered within 49 months and costs associated with laparoscopic surgery can be recovered as early as 25 months post-surgery.

No definitive conclusion can yet be drawn on the cost effectiveness of each bariatric operation. Roux-en-Y gastric bypass and adjustable gastric banding both are cost effective with incremental cost effectiveness ratios of $25,000 per quality adjusted life years. Adjustable gastric banding is relatively more cost effective over shorter periods of time in diabetic obese patients. However costs associated with band fills impact negatively on cost effectiveness. Dominance of any one procedure over the other also appears to depend on the region and patient selection.

After including the indirect economic impact of bariatric surgery on workers' productivity along with the direct impact on health services, the overall economic effectiveness of bariatric surgery may become even more significant.

Abbreviations

AGB	Adjustable gastric band
AUD	Australian dollar
BMI	Body mass index
CEA	Cost effectiveness analysis
DM	Diabetes mellitus
GERD	Gastroesophageal reflux disease
HSE	Health Survey for England
HTN	Hypertension
ICER	Incremental cost effectiveness ratio
ICUR	Incremental cost utility ratio
MEPS	Medical Expenditure Panel Survey
NHWS	National Health and Wellness Survey
NHS	National Health Service
RCT	Randomised controlled trial
RYGB	Roux-en-Y gastric bypass
QALY	Quality adjusted life year
VBG	Vertical banded gastroplasty

References

Abell, T.L., Minocha, A. (2006). Gastrointestinal complications of bariatric surgery: diagnosis and therapy. Am. J. Med. Sci. 2006; 331(4):214–8

Ackroyd, R., Mouiel, J., Chevallier, J., Daoud, F. (2006). Cost-Effectiveness and Budget Impact of Obesity Surgery in Patients With Type-2 Diabetes in Three European Countries. Obes Surg. 2006; 16(11):1488–1503

Anselmino, M., Bammer, T., Cebrián, J.M.F. (2009). Cost-effectiveness and Budget Impact of Obesity Surgery in Patients with Type 2 Diabetes in Three European Countries (II). Obes Surg. 2009; 19(11):1542–1549

Ashrafian, H., le Roux, C.W., Darzi, A., Athanasiou, T. (2008). Effects of bariatric surgery on cardiovascular function. Circulation. 2008; 118(20):2091–102

Buchwald, H., Avidor, Y., Braunwald, E., et al. (2004). Bariatric surgery: a systematic review and meta-analysis. JAMA. 2004; 292(14):1724–37

Butland, B., Jebb, S., Kopelman, P., et al. (2007). Tackling Obesities: Future Choices – Project Report (2nd Ed). London: Foresight Programme of the Government Office for Science, 2007. Available at: https://www.gov.uk/government/uploads/system/uploads/attachment_data/file/287937/07-1184x-tackling-obesities-future-choices-report.pdf

Campbell, J., McGarry, L.J., Shikora, S.A., et al. (2010). Cost-Effectiveness of Laparoscopic Gastric Banding and Bypass for Morbid Obesity. Am J Manag Care. 2010; 16(7):e174–e187

Clinical Guidelines on the Identification, Evaluation, and Treatment of Overweight and Obesity in Adults: The Evidence Report. 1998. [Accessed: 7 July 2014.] Available at: http://www.nhlbi.nih.gov/files/docs/guidelines/ob_gdlns.pdf

Craig, B.M., Tseng, D.S. (2002). Cost-effectiveness of gastric bypass for severe obesity. Am J Med. 2002; 113(6):491–498

Crémieux, P., Buchwald, H., Shikora, S.A., et al. (2008). A Study on the Economic Impact of Bariatric Surgery. Am J Manag Care. 2008; 14(9):589–596

Dumon, K.R., Murayam, K.M. (2011). Bariatric surgery outcomes. Surgical Clinics of North America. 2011; 91(6):1313–1338

Elder, K.A., Wolfe, B.M. (2007). Bariatric Surgery: A Review of Procedures and Outcomes. Gastroenterology. 2007; 132(6):2253–2271

Ewing, B.T., Thompson, M.A., Wachtel, M.S., Frezza, E.E. (2001). A cost-benefit analysis of bariatric surgery on the South Plains region of Texas. Obes Surg. 2001; 21(5):644–9

Finkelstein, E.A., Allaire, B.T., Burgess, S., Hale, B.C. (2011). Financial implications of coverage for laparoscopic adjustable gastric banding. Surg Obes Relat Dis. 2011; 7(3):295–303

Finkelstein, E.A., Allaire, B.T., DiBonaventura, M, Burgess, S. (2011). Direct and Indirect Costs and Potential Cost Savings of Laparoscopic Adjustable Gastric Banding Among Obese Patients With Diabetes. J Occup Environ Med. 2011; 53(9):1025–9

Goodell, S, Cohen, J., Neumann, P. (2009). Policy Cost savings and cost-effectiveness of clinical preventative care. The Synthesis Project. Brief No. 18. Robert Wood Johnson Foundation. 2009. Available at: http://www.rwjf.org/content/dam/supplementary-assets/2009/09/Cost-Savings-and-Cost-Effectiveness-Clinical-Preventive-Care-Brief.pdf

Haslam, D.W., James, W.P. (2005). Obesity. Lancet. 2005; 366(9492):1197–1209

Hawkins, S.C., Osborne, A., Finlay, I.G., et al. (2007). Paid work increases and state benefit claims decrease after bariatric surgery. Obes Surg. 2007; 17(4):434–437

Hayashi, S.Y., Faintuch, J., França, J.I.D., Cecconello, I. (2011). Four-Year Hospital Resource Utilization After Bariatric Surgery: Comparison with Clinical and Surgical Controls. Obes Surg. 2011; 21(9):1355–1361

Hoerger, T.J., Zhang, P., Segel, J.E., et al. (2010). Cost-Effectiveness of Bariatric Surgery for Severely Obese Adults With Diabetes. Diabetes Care. 2010; 33(9):1933–1939

Hutter, M.M., Randall, S., Khuri, S.F., et al. (2006). Laparoscopic Versus Open Gastric Bypass for Morbid Obesity. Ann Surg. 2006; 243(5): 657–666

Ikramuddin, S., Klingman, C.D., Swan, T., Minshall, M.E. (2009). Cost-Effectiveness of Roux-en-Y Gastric Bypass in Type 2 Diabetes Patients. Am J Manag Care. 2009; 15(9):607–615

Keating, C.L., Dixon, J.B., Moodie, M.L., et al. (2009). Cost-Effectiveness of Surgically Induced Weight Loss for the Management of Type 2 Diabetes: Modelled Lifetime Analysis. Diabetes Care. 2009; 32(4):567–574

Keating, C.L., Dixon, J.B., Moodie, M.L., et al. (2009). Cost-Efficacy of Surgically Induced Weight Loss for the Management of Type 2 Diabetes. Diabetes Care. 2009; 32(4):580–4

Maciejewski, M.L,. Smith, V.A., Livingston, E.H., et al. (2010). Health Care Utilization and Expenditure Changes Associated With Bariatric Surgery. Med Care. 2010; 48(11): 989–998

Maggard, M.A., Shugarman, L.R., Suttorp, M., et al. (2005). Meta-analysis: surgical treatment of obesity. Ann Intern Med. 2005; 142(7):547–59

Makary, M.A., Clark, J.M., Shore, A.D., et al. (2010). Medication utilization and annual health care costs in patients with type 2 diabetes mellitus before and after bariatric surgery. Arch Surg. 2010; 145(8):726–31

Maklin, S., Malmivaara, A., Linna, M., et al. (2011). Cost–utility of bariatric surgery for morbid obesity in Finland. Br J Surg. 2011; 98:1422–1429

McEwen, L.N., Coelho, R.B., Baumann, L.M., et al. (2010). The Cost, Quality of Life Impact, and Cost–Utility of Bariatric Surgery in a Managed Care Population. Obes Surg. 2010; 20(7):919–928

Mullen, D.M., Marr, T.J. (2010). Longitudinal cost experience for gastric bypass patients. Surg Obes Relat Dis. 2010; 6:243–248

National Obesity Observatory. (2014). Public Health England: Adult obesity and type 2 diabetes. 2014.. Available at: http://www.noo.org.uk/securefiles/140915_1106/Adult_obesity_and_type_2_diabetes_20140730.pdf

Nguyen, N.T., Goldman, C., Rosenquist, C.J., et al. (2001). Laparoscopic versus open gastric bypass: a randomized study of outcomes, quality of life, and costs. Ann Surg. 2001; 234(3):279–89

Nguyen, N.T., Slone, J.A., Nguyen, X.T., et al. (2009). A Prospective Randomized Trial of Laparoscopic Gastric Bypass Versus Laparoscopic Adjustable Gastric Banding for the Treatment of Morbid Obesity; Outcomes, Quality of Life, and Costs. Ann Surg. 2009; 250:631–641

Nguyen, N.T., Varela, E., Sabio, A., et al. (2006). Reduction in prescription medication costs after laparoscopic gastric bypass. The American Surgeon. 2006; 72(10):853–856

Ojo, P., Valin, E. (2009). Cost-Effective Restrictive Bariatric Surgery: Laparoscopic Vertical Banded Gastroplasty Versus Laparoscopic Adjustable Gastric Band. Obes Surg. 2009; 19:1536–1541

Palmer, S., Byford S., Raftery, J., (1999). Types of economic evaluation BMJ.1999;318(7194): 1349

Reoch, J., Mottillo, S., Shimony, A., et al. (2011). Safety of laparoscopic vs open bariatric surgery: a systematic review and meta-analysis. Arch Surg. 2011; 146(11):1314–22

Salem, L., Devlin, A., Sullivan, S.D., Flum, D.R. (2008). A cost-effectiveness analysis of laparoscopic gastric bypass, adjustable gastric banding, and non-surgical weight loss interventions. Surg Obes Relat Dis. 2008; 4(1):26–32

Sampalis, J.S., Liberman, M., Auger, S., Christou, N.V. (2004) The Impact of Weight Reduction Surgery on Health-Care Costs in Morbidly Obese Patients. Obes Surg. 2004; 14(7):939–947

Shabbir, A., Loi, T.H., Lomanto, D., Ti, T.K., So, J.B. (2009). Surgical Management of Obesity – National University Hospital Experience. Ann Acad Med Singapore. 2009; 38(10):882–90

Sjöström, L., Lindroos, A.K., Peltonen, M., et al. (2004). Lifestyle, diabetes, and cardiovascular risk factors 10 years after bariatric surgery. N Engl J Med. 2004; 351(26):2683–93

Sjöström, L., Peltonen, M., Jacobson, P., et al. (2012). Bariatric surgery and long-term cardiovascular events. JAMA. 2012; 307(1):56–65

Stanczyk, M., Martindale, R.G., Deveney, C. (2007). "53 Bariatric Surgery Overview". In C.D. Berdanier, E.B. Feldman, J. Dwyer. Handbook of Nutrition and Food. Boca Raton, FL: CRC Press. pp. 915–926

van Gemert, W.G., Adang, E.M., Kop, M., et al. (1999). A Prospective Cost-Effectiveness Analysis of Vertical Banded Gastroplasty for the Treatment of Morbid Obesity. Obes Surg. 1999; 9(5):484–91

Waxman, K.T. (2013). Financial and Business Management for the Doctor of Nursing Practice pg 185, 2013 Springer publishing Company

Chapter 4

Use of Biologics for Management of Rheumatoid Arthritis

Canna Ghia[1], Jignesh Ved[1], Gautam Rambhad[1]

1 Introduction

Rheumatoid arthritis (RA) is a chronic, frequently progressive, and destructive autoimmune disease. As the disease progresses, irreversible joint damage may lead to loss of function and physical disability (World Health Organization, 2004). Patients with RA have reduced quality of life compared with healthy people. RA is associated with serious co-morbidities such as heart disease, infection, and malignancies (Boonen & Severens, 2011). This can result in a 5–10 year reduction in life expectancy (Kvien, 2004), reduced quality of life compared with other serious conditions (Lundkvist *et al.*, 2008) and a considerable economic burden (Lundkvist *et al.*, 2008). RA is a disabling disease, and the disability is usually measured by using a questionnaire called the Health Assessment Questionnaire (HAQ). Assement of Assessment for tenderness and swelling in the joints is one by the DAS (Disease Activity Score) for 28 joints. The counting of number of swollen and tender joints in the following 28-joints is done: 10 proximal interphalangeal joints (PIP), 10 metacarpo-phalangeal joints (MCP), 2 wrists, 2 elbows, 2 shoulders and 2 knees (Misra *et al.*, 2008).

Since this disease cannot be cured, management of this disease becomes an important endeavor with the aim of inducing and maintaining remission, and altering the course of disease. Disease Modifying AntiRheumatic Drugs (DMARDs, methotrexate followed by leflunoamide, sulfasalazine and hydroxychloroquine) are the recommended first line treatment for RA. However they are slow acting and toxicity monitoring is essential in patients on DMARDs ("Indian Guidelines", 2002; Misra *et al.*, 2008) Corticosteroids are affordable and do have a disease modifying effect, but are beneficial when

---

[1] Medical and Research Department, Pfizer Limited, India

used over a short period of time, beyond this side effects outweigh any benefit. Routine use of steroids is therefore not recommended (Misra *et al.*, 2008). Other drugs like Non-steroidal anti-inflammatory drugs (NSAIDs), gold salts, hydroxychloroquine, d-penicillamine are also used in the treatment but have varied effects (Misra *et al.*, 2008).

The approach to treatment of RA has seen significant advances in the last two decades. There has been a paradigm shift in the management of RA which now aims at induction of remission and maintenance of tight control (treat to target) through use of conventional DMARDs and biologics therapy. Biological agents that target inflammatory cytokines and cells within the synovium and immune system are now widely available. Biologics approved for RA include abatacept, adalimumab, anakinra, etanercept, infliximab, golimumab, rituximab and tocilizumab. These agents not only reduce the signs and symptoms but also slow down the progression of the disease. Despite their clinical superiority, biologics can cause side effects (pain at injection site, infusion reaction, chances of super infection and reactivation of tubercular bacteria in some cases) and do not work in some patients.

The use of biologics has consolidated the management of RA. Debate still exists as to when one should start biologics, how long they should be used, how they should be tapered off, whether one biologic can be switched with another. This review focuses on available biologics, their differences, clinical considerations for biological therapy in RA, the advent of biosimilars/intended copies in the space of RA, data from biologic registries and the future perspectives in RA treatment.

1.1   Historical Background

These agents are called biologics because they mimic the action of proteins involved in the immune system, these agents did bring about a greater relief to patients than any other treatment known and hence the real excitement in rheumatology happened after the introduction of these biological agents in 1998. They are made by genetic engineering in tissue cultures of various kinds. The work in the arena of biologics in RA started way back in the late 1980s when tumor necrosis factor-alpha (TNF-*a*) was identified in the synovium of RA patients (Buchan *et al.*, 1988). Specific antibody to block this TNF-*a* (CA2) was simultaneously produced. This CA2 was a chimeric-mouse human antibody (later named infliximab). Initially CA2 was used as a tool for the further determination of importance of TNF-*a* in the pathogenesis of RA. Experiments showed that synovial membrane cells produced a number of inflammatory molecules including the cytokines TNF-*a* and interleukin-1 (IL-1) (Breenan *et al.*, 1989; Feldmann *et al.*, 1990). When TNF –*a* was blocked using antibodies like CA2 it appeared that it had a unique position in the hierarchy of inflammatory cytokines. Blocking TNF-*a* also blocked the production of other cytokines, including IL-1 (Feldmann *et al.*, 1990). Follow up experiments demonstrated the efficacy of TNF-*a* blockade in animal models of RA (Williams *et al.*, 1992). A very successful pilot study in the early 1990s showed that TNF-*a* blocking antibodies administered intravenously to human subjects with RA showed dramatic results (Elliot *et al.*, 1993). In an effort to reduce the risk of immunogenicity as much as possible, further development has led the production of fully human antibodies that contain 100% human protein. Adalimumab was the first fully human recombinant anti-TNF-a monoclonal antibody (mAb) approved for the treatment of patients with RA (Bain & Brazil, 2003). Other biologics (etanercept, rituximab, abatacept, anakinra, golimumab and abatacept) also made their way in the RA management armamentarium.

2   Biological Agents in RA

The introduction of "biological agents" has revolutionized the treatment of RA. These therapies target pro-inflammatory cytokines (e.g. TNF-a, IL-1 or IL-6) or cellular membrane receptors (e.g. CD20 and CD4) in the sufferers (Fan & Leong, 2007). All these agents have been evaluated against the ACR 20, ACR50 and ACR70 outcomes, European League Against Rheumatism (EULAR) response criteria based on the Disease Activity Score (DAS) on 28- or 44-joint count were also adopted and the Health Assessment allowed for the accurate assessment of functional status.

Biologic	Approved Year	Class	Type	Target
Infliximab	1998	Chimeric mAb	IgG1	TNF-a
Etanercept	1998	Human dimeric fusion protein	Fusion protein	TNF-a; TNF-B (lymphotoxin a)
Anakinra	2001	Human interleukin-1 receptor antagonist	Receptor antagonist	IL-1
Adalimumab	2002	Human mAb	IgG1	TNF-a
Abatacept	2005	Human dimeric fusion protein	Fusion protein	CD-28
Rituximab	2006	Chimeric mAb	IgG1	CD-20
Certolizumab pegol	2008	Humanized mAb	Fab	TNF-a
Golimumab	2009	Human mAb	IgG1	TNF-a
Tocilizumab	2009	Humanized mAb	IgG1	IL-6R

Table 1: Lists the biologics approved in RA worldwide.

2.1   Monoclonal Antibodies in RA

2.1.1   Infliximab

- **Indications** In combination with methotrexate (MTX) for the treatment of RA in patients who have had an inadequate response to MTX alone. It is also indicated for the treatment of active, severe RA patients' naïve for MTX or other disease modifying antirheumatic drugs (DMARDs), Crohn's disease, ankylosing spondylitis, psoriatic arthritis, ulcerative colitis and plaque psoriasis.

- **Structure** Chimeric IgG1 mAb, with murine variable (Fv) domain of mouse anti-human TNF-*a* antibody and constant (Fc) sequences of human IgG1, produced by recombinant cell culture technique.

- **Mechanism of action**   Specifically recognizes and binds with both soluble and membrane-bound TNF-*a*. This binding neutralizes the biological activity of TNF-*a* by inhibiting its binding to receptor (Scallon *et al.*, 1995). By blocking TNF-*a*, infliximab reduces the release of pro-inflammatory cytokines (IL-1 and IL-6) and acute phase reactants, the activation of eosinophils and neutrophils, and the leucocyte migration (Janssen Biotech Inc, 2013a). Infliximab does not neutralize TNF-*B* (lymphotoxin a).

- **Dosage** Infliximab is usually given as a 3 mg/kg dose by intravenous (IV) infusion to RA patients followed by similar doses at 2 and 6 weeks after the first infusion, then every 8 weeks, although the dose can be increased up to 7.5 mg/kg. It should be administered in combination with methotrexate (MTX).

- **Adverse events** Severe side effects are rare; however, the chances of tuberculosis (TB) are highly increased in patients receiving infliximab (Gardam *et al.*, 2003) and therefore treatment of latent TB infection is recommended, prior to initiating the therapy (Janssen Biotech Inc, 2013a). The most common adverse events are headache, vertigo, viral infection, flushing, upper and lower respiratory tract infection, (Janssen Biotech Inc, 2013a).

- **Clinical efficacy** In RA patients whose disease remains active despite MTX, infliximab, in combination with MTX, has been shown to reduce signs and symptoms, to inhibit radiographic progression of structural damage and to improve physical function in RA patients not responding to MTX. The three multicentre phase III clinical trials termed ATTRACT (Anti- TNF Trial in Rheumatoid Arthritis with Concomitant Therapy) (Gardam *et al.*, 2003), ASPIRE (Active-controlled Study of Patients receiving Infliximab for treatment of Rheumatoid arthritis of Early onset) (Lipsky *et al.*, 2000) and START (Safety Trial for Rheumatoid Arthritis with Remicade [infliximab] Therapy) (St. Clair *et al.*, 2004; Westhovens *et al.*, 2006) done in around 2500 RA patients does justify this. Herein ACR20 was reached by a 1.5- to 3-fold higher patient rate with infliximab than placebo. Radiographic progression was reduced not only in patients in the ATTRACT study who had a clinical response to infliximab plus MTX, but also in those who did not have a clinical response (Smolen *et al.*, 2005).

2.1.2   Adalimumab

- **Indications** For RA in combination with MTX, in patients who have had an inadequate response to MTX alone. For the treatment of active, severe RA patients naïve for MTX or other DMARDs, psoriatic arthritis, ankylosing spondylitis, plaque psoriasis, juvenile idiopathic arthritis, Crohn's disease, ulcerative colitis and non-radiographic axial spondyloarthritis.

- **Structure** Adalimumab is a recombinant fully human monoclonal IgG1 antibody, composed of two kappa light chains (24 kDa each) and two IgG1 heavy chains (49 kDa each), expressed in Chinese hamster ovary (CHO) cells. Because of human origin it is less immunogenic than infliximab (Paul & Anderson, 2005)

- **Mechanism of action** Adalimumab recognizes both soluble and membrane-bound TNF-*a* and inhibits its biologic activity by blocking interaction with p55 and p75 cell surface TNFR1 and TNFR2 receptors (Rau, 2002). Furthermore, adalimumab treatment exerts the down regulation of expression of other pro-inflammatory cytokines, such as IL-6, IL-8 and GM-CSF (granulocyte macrophage colony-stimulating factor) (AbbVie Inc, 2014).

- **Dosage** For adult RA patients, the recommended dose is 40 mg on every other week, as a subcutaneous injection. It can be administered in combination with MTX or as monotherapy

- **Adverse events** Because adalimumab is a fully human antibody, some potential adverse reactions and antigenicity of chimeric and humanized mAbs should be minimized. However, like infliximab, the chances of TB infection reactivation are highly increased in patients receiving adalimumab; therefore, treatment of latent TB infection is mandatory, prior to initiating the therapy (AbbVie Inc, 2014). Most common side effects are injection site reaction, upper respiratory infection, sinusitis, leucopenia, anaemia, hyperlipidaemia,and so on. The production of anti-adalimumab antibodies (AAA) has also been seen in clinical trials in patients with RA (AbbVie Inc, 2014).

- **Clinical efficacy** In patients with active RA the addition of adalimumab to long-term MTX therapy provided significant, rapid and sustained improvement in disease activity over 24 weeks compared with MTX plus placebo, as shown by the ARMADA (Anti-TNF Research study program of the Monoclonal Antibody D2E7 in patients with Rheumatoid Arthritis) trial (Weinblatt *et al.*, 2003). The long-term, open label extension of this clinical trial demonstrated that adalimumab plus MTX was associated with sustained clinical response and remission in patients with RA over a 4-year period (Weinblatt, 2006). The PREMIER study, conducted at 133 investigational sites across the world showed that in patients with early, aggressive RA, combination therapy with adalimumab plus MTX was significantly superior to either MTX or adalimumab monotherapy in improving signs and symptoms of disease, inhibiting radiographic progression and reaching clinical remission (Breedveld *et al*, 2006). Moreover the ReAct (Research in Active Rheumatoid Arthritis trial) recently demonstrated that adalimumab induced a good clinical response after 12 weeks of treatment in 69 % of patients who failed with other biologic or non-biologic DMARDs (Burmester *et al.*, 2007).

2.1.3   Rituximab

- **Indications** For the treatment of patients with moderately to severely active RA who did not adequately respond to one or more TNF antagonist therapies

- **Structure** Rituximab is a genetically engineered chimeric murine/human monoclonal antibody to CD20 antigen found on the surface of normal and malignant B lymphocytes. It is produced by a cell suspension culture technique in a CHO cell mammalian expression system. The rituximab antibody consists of IgG1 kappa Ig containing variable region sequences of murine light chains (213 amino acids) and heavy chains (451 amino acids) and human constant region sequences (Biogen Idec Inc, 2014).

- **Mechanism of action** CD20 is a B cell-specific antigen expressed on the surface of B lymphocytes. Rituximab is a monoclonal antibody that targets the CD20 antigen expressed on the surface of pre-B and mature B-lymphocytes. Upon binding to CD20, rituximab mediates B-cell lysis. Possible mechanisms of cell lysis include complement dependent cytotoxicity (CDC) and antibody dependent cell mediated cytotoxicity (ADCC). The antibody induced apoptosis in the DHL 4 human B cell lymphoma cell line. B cells are believed to play a role in the pathogenesis of RA and associated chronic synovitis. In this setting, B cells may be acting at multiple sites in the autoimmune/inflammatory process, including through production of rheumatoid factor (RF) and other autoantibodies, antigen presentation, T-cell activation, and/or proinflammatory cytokine production (Stern & Hermann *et al*, 2005).

- **Dosage** In RA rituximab is given as two 1,000 mg i.v. infusions separated by 2 weeks

- **Adverse events** Common adverse events reported are infections which include upper respiratory tract infections, bronchitis, nasopharyngitis, sinusitis and urinary tract infections. The incidence of serious infections in the rituximab-treated patients was 2 versus 1 % in the placebo treated patients (Biogen Idec Inc, 2014).

- **Clinical efficacy** In patients with active RA despite MTX treatment, a single course of two infusions of rituximab (1,000 mg on days 1 and 15), alone or in combination with either cyclophosphamide or MTX, provided significant improvement in disease symptoms at both weeks 24 and 48 (Olszewski & Grossbard, 2004). A phase III study on 520 RA patients demonstrated that a single course of two 1,000 mg infusions of rituximab administered 2 weeks apart, in combination with glucocorticoids and MTX, produced significant clinical and functional benefits at 24 weeks in patients with longstanding and active RA who had an inadequate response to one or more anti-TNF-*a* therapies (Edwards *et al.*, 2004).

2.1.4   Tocilizumab

- **Indications** For the treatment of patients with moderate to severe active RA who do not respond to one or more DMARDs or TNF antagonist therapies

- **Structure** Tocilizumab is a humanized anti-human IL-6R antibody engineered by grafting the complementarity determining regions (CDRs) of a mouse anti-human

IL-6R antibody into human IgG1 to create a humanized mAb with a human IL-6R specificity (Sato *et al.*, 1993).

- **Mechanism of action** IL-6 is a pro-inflammatory cytokine that binds specifically to both soluble and membrane-bound IL-6 receptors (sIL-6R and mIL-6R) and Tocilizumab inhibits sIL-6R and mIL-6R-mediated signaling. Thus it entirely neutralizes IL-6 actions (Sato *et al.*, 1993).

- **Dosage** Dosage is 8 mg per kg of body weight, once every 4 weeks intravenously; however, depending on the patient's response, the physician may decrease the dose when appropriate. There is no reported experience with the use of tocilizumab with TNF antagonists and/or other biologic treatments for RA; therefore, at the moment it is not recommended for use with other biological therapies. Tocilizumab can be used subcutaneously also.

- **Adverse events** Upper respiratory tract infections are very common adverse events of tocilizumab; Common adverse reactions may include lung infection (pneumonia), abnormal liver function tests, conjunctivitis, headache, hypertension and serious hypersensitivity reactions

- **Clinical efficacy** Three multicentre, double-blind, placebo-controlled phase III trials evaluated the efficacy and safety of tocilizumab. In the OPTION (tOcilizumab Pivotal Trial in methotrexate Inadequate respONders) trial, 59 and 48 % of 623 patients who received tocilizumab 8 and 4 mg/kg plus MTX, respectively, achieved ACR20 at week 24, compared with 27 % of patients who received placebo plus MTX (Smolen *et al.*, 2008). The TOWARD (Tocilizumab in cOmbination With traditional DMARD therapy) trial found that 61 % of 805 patients who received tocilizumab 8 mg/kg plus DMARD(s) achieved ACR20 at week 24, compared with 25 % of 415 patients treated with DMARDs plus placebo (Genovese *et al.*, 2008). LITHE trial (tociLIzumab safety and THE prevention of structural joint damage) showed in 1,196 patients followed for 2 years an improvement in disease activity or disease remission (DAS28- Diseaase activity score of 28 joints- 2.6) in 30 and 47 % of patients treated with tocilizumab 4 and 8 mg/kg, respectively, compared with 8 % of patients treated with placebo plus MTX. Additionally, the 1-year LITHE study results showed that patients treated with tocilizumab (4 or 8 mg/kg) plus MTX experienced a significant inhibition in the progression of structural joint damage, as measured by the change in the mean Genant-modified Sharp score, compared with patients treated with MTX plus placebo (Kremer *et al*, 2009).

2.1.5   Golimumab

- **Indications** For the treatment of moderate to severe active RA, in combination with MTX, in patients who have had an inadequate response to MTX alone. It is also indicated for the treatment of active, severe RA patients naive for MTX or other DMARDs, active and progressive psoriatic arthritis and severe, active ankylosing spondylitis.

- **Structure** Golimumab is a fully human IgG1 monoclonal antibody against TNF-*a* that targets and neutralizes both the soluble and the membrane-bound form of TNF-*a* (Hirohata *et al.*, 2007).

- **Mechanism of action** Golimumab binds with high affinity to both the soluble and transmembrane forms of TNF-*a*. It forms large complexes when bound to TNF-*a* trimers, usually three golimumab molecules bind to one or two TNF-*a* trimers. The binding of golimumab with human TNF-*a* inhibits the binding of TNF-*a* to p55 and p75 TNF-a receptor fusion protein, and neutralizes TNF-*a*-induced cell-surface expression of the adhesion molecule E-selectin, vascular cell adhesion molecule (VCAM-1) and intercellular adhesion molecule (ICAM-1) by human endothelial cells. Golimumab does not bind with human lymphotoxin(Hirohata *et al.*, 2007; Janssen Biotech Inc, 2013b).

- **Dosage** Golimumab is administered subcutaneously every 4 weeks. It is given in a single 50-mg dose, via a prefilled autoinjector or prefilled syringe; however, this dose could be doubled if the patient has a body weight of more than 100 kg and has no response after 3–4 doses (Janssen Biotech Inc, 2013b).

- **Adverse events** Mild to severe bacterial, viral and other infections along with anemia, headache, allergic reactions (bronchospasm, hypersensitivity, urticaria), increase in liver enzymes, constipation, abdominal pain, dyspepsia, hypertension, and so on have been reported(Janssen Biotech Inc, 2013b).

- **Clinical efficacy** Golimumab has been studied for the treatment of moderate to severe active RA in multicentre, randomized, double-blind controlled trials that enrolled over 1,500 patients. These trials were called GO-FORWARD, in which enrolled RA patients naïve for biologic TNF-a blocker (*N* = 444) had active RA despite a stable dosage of at least 15 mg/week of MTX (Keystone *et al.*, 2008a) ; GO-AFTER, in which enrolled RA patients were previously treated with one or more anti-TNF-*a* agents (*N* = 461) (Smolen *et al.*, 2009a); and GO-BEFORE, which enrolled patients with active RA who were MTX-naïve (*N* = 637) (Emery *et al.*, 2009). In these studies golimumab was shown to improve signs and symptoms in moderate to severe active RA patients. It has been shown to be effective in RA patients who are incomplete responders or naive to MTX, as well as in those patients previously treated with at least one anti-TNF-*a* therapy.

2.1.6   Certolizumab Pegol

- **Indications** For the treatment of adults with moderate to severe active RA in combination with MTX, in patients who have had an inadequate response to MTX alone.

- **Structure** Certolizumab pegol is a recombinant, humanized anti-TNF-*a* Fab conjugated to approximately 40,000 Da polyethylene glycol (PEG2-MAL40K) (Winter *et al.*, 2004). The Fab is manufactured in Escherichia coli and is subsequently purified and conjugated to PEG2MAL40K, to produce certolizumab pegol.

- **Mechanism of action** Certolizumab pegol binds to human TNF-a with high affinity and neutralizes both membrane-bound and soluble forms. It does not neutralize lymphotoxin a (TNF-*B*) (Nesbitt & Henry, 2004).

- **Dosage** The recommended dosage of certolizumab pegol for adult RA patients is 400 mg (given as two subcutaneous injections of 200 mg) initially and at weeks 2 and 4, followed by 200 mg every other week. However, for maintenance dosing 400 mg every 4 weeks can be considered.

- **Adverse events** Viral and bacterial infections have been commonly reported.Other common adverse events are headache, allergic reactions (bronchospasm, hypersensitivity and urticaria), increase in liver enzymes, rash, pyrexia, leucopenia, pain, and so on

- **Clinical efficacy** Phase III FAST4WARD (eFficAcy and Safety of cerTolizumab pegol – 4 Weekly dosAge in RheumatoiD arthritis) study demonstrated that treatment with certolizumab pegol 400 mg monotherapy every 4 weeks effectively reduced the signs and symptoms of active RA in patients previously failing more than one DMARD compared with placebo, and demonstrated an acceptable safety profile (Fleischmann *et al.*, 2009). In the RAPID 1 and 2 (Rheumatoid Arthritis PreventIon of structural Damage) studies conducted on over 1,600 active RA patients, certolizumab pegol allowed patients to reach ACR20, 50 or 70 in a 3- to 15-fold higher patient percentage than placebo (Smolen *et al.*, 2009b; Keystone *et al.*, 2008b).

2.2   Fusion Proteins in RA

2.2.1   Abatacept

- **Indications** For the treatment of patients with moderate to severe active RA who had inadequate response to one or more DMARDs, including MTX and TNF-*a* antagonists (Moreland *et al.*, 2006). Also indicated in patients with moderate to severe juvenile idiopathic arthritis (JIA) who had inadequate response to other DMARDs, including at least one TNF antagonist and in adult RA naive to TNF-*a* inhibitors. Abatacept may be used as a monotherapy or concomitantly with DMARDs.

- **Structure** Abatacept is a fully human soluble fusion protein comprising the extracellular domain of human cytotoxic T lymphocyte associated antigen-4 (CTLA-4) linked to the Fc (hinge, CH2 and CH3 domains) portion of human IgG1.

- **Mechanism of action** T cells require two distinct signals for full activation. The first signal is an antigen-specific interaction between the antigenic peptide presented in the context of the major histocompatibility complex (MHC) on the surface of antigen-presenting cells (APC) and the T cell receptor. The second signal comes from the binding of a ligand on the APC to the co-stimulatory receptor on the T cell; the interaction of CD28 on T cells with CD80 or CD86 on APCs is a key example of a costimulatory signal (Linsley *et al.*, 1992). CTLA-4 instead is the inhibitory CD28 counterpart. Abatacept binds with its extracellular CTLA-4 portion to CD80 and CD86 on APC with a higher affinity than CD28, thus blocking its interaction with CD28 on T cells (Linsley *et al.*, 1992). Therefore, abatacept prevents the positive co-stimulation signal required for full T cell activation.

- **Dosage** Recommended dose is 10 mg/kg of body weight. For an adult patient with body weight below 60 kg the recommended dose is 500 mg, for 61–100 kg it is 750 mg and for over 100 kg it is 1,000 mg; following the initial administration, abatacept should be given at 2 and 4 weeks after the first infusion and every 4 weeks thereafter. Abatacept can be used subcutaneously also.

- **Adverse events** Most common side effects with abatacept are upper respiratory infections, including nasopharyngitis. Moreover, lower respiratory tract infections, urinary tract infections, leucopenia, headache, conjunctivitis, arterial hypertension, cough, abdominal pain, diarrhoea, nausea, vomiting, dyspepsia, increase of liver enzymes, rash, alopecia, itching, arthralgia and asthenia may also commonly be observed. (Bristol-Myers Squibb Company, 2013; Weinblatt *et al.*, 2006)

- **Clinical efficacy** The AIM (Abatacept in Inadequate responders to Methotrexate) study, a 12-month, double-blind, randomized, placebo-controlled investigation on 638 RA patients, demonstrated that combination of abatacept and MTX improved the signs and symptoms of disease, physical function and quality of life in patients who had active RA despite ongoing MTX therapy. Clinical responses were dose-dependent; patients treated with 10 mg of abatacept per kg achieved the best results. Abatacept was safe and well tolerated, and the rate of discontinuation because of adverse events was no higher than that in the placebo group (Reiser & Stadecker, 1996). A further phase III trial called ATTAIN (Abatacept Trial in Treatment of Anti-TNF INadequate responders) of 6-month duration in RA patients with a current or previous inadequate response to TNF-*a* inhibitors therapy also demonstrated significant benefit with abatacept in this patient population (Emery *et al.*, 2006). ASSURE (Abatacept Study of Safety in Use with other RA thErapies) studied the safety of abatacept compared to placebo when used in combination with biologic and nonbiologic DMARDs (Weinblatt *et al.*, 2006).

2.2.2   Etanercept

- **Indications** In combination with MTX for moderate to severe active RA and juvenile idiopathic arthritis. It is also indicated for ankylosing spondylitis, psoriatic and chronic plaque psoriasis including pediatric psoriasis

- **Structure** Etanercept is a fully human dimeric fusion protein, produced by recombinant DNA technology in a CHO mammalian cell expression system. It consists of two molecules, the extracellular portion of soluble TNFR2 (p75) receptor and the constant (Fc) portion of an IgG1 heavy chain (Feldman & Maini, 2001). The Fc component contains the CH2 domain, the CH3 domain and hinge region, but not the CH1 domain of IgG1 (Immunex Corporation, 2013).

- **Mechanism of action** Etanercept is a competitive inhibitor of the binding of TNF-*a* to its cell surface receptor and can bind to two TNF molecules. It inhibits the biological function of TNF-*a* by preventing the receptor stimulation. It binds primarily to soluble TNF-a as well as TNF-*B* (lymphotoxin-*a*) by cell surface TNFRs (Feldman & Maini, 2001; Immunex Corporation, 2013).

- **Dosage** Recommended dosage is 50 mg given once a week. MTX, salicylates, glucocorticoids, non-steroidal anti-inflammatory drugs (NSAIDs) or analgesics may be continued during treatment.

- **Adverse events** Common side effects include injection site reactions, upper and lower respiratory infections, urinary tract and skin infections, allergic reactions,and so on (Feldman & Maini, 2001; Immunex Corporation, 2013)..

- **Clinical efficacy** In patients with early, active RA etanercept as monotherapy slowed radiographic progression, and improved the disability index score significantly better than MTX monotherapy did over a 2-year period (Genovese *et al.*, 2002). The TEMPO (Trial of Etanercept and Methotrexate with radiographic and Patient Outcomes) study compared the combination of etanercept and MTX with either etanercept or MTX monotherapy in patients with active RA in whom previous treatment with DMARDs other than MTX had failed. The 2-year data demonstrated that combination therapy was significantly better than either monotherapy in reducing disease activity, improving function and slowing radiographic progression (van der Heijde *et al.*, 2006). The COMET (COmbination of Methotrexate and ETanercept in early rheumatoid arthritis) study compared the clinical efficacy and safety of etanercept and methotrexate combination therapy with methotrexate alone on clinical disease activity and progressive joint damage in patients with early active RA. According to 2-year results from this trial treating RA patients with a combination of etanercept plus methotrexate leads to better results (gives better performance) than methotrexate alone (Emery *et al.*, 2008).

2.3   Receptor Antagonists for Treatment of RA

2.3.1   Anakinra

- **Indications** For RA patients who have failed one or more DMARDs.

- **Structure** Anakinra is a recombinant, nonglycosylated form of the human interleukin-1 receptor antagonist (IL-1ra), which is produced in E. coli expression systems by recombinant DNA technology (Calabrese,2002; Arend, 2002).

- **Mechanism of action** Anakinra blocks the biologic activity of interleukin-1a (IL-1a) and interleukin-1b (IL-1b) by competitively inhibiting their binding to interleukin- 1 type I receptor (IL-1RI). IL-1 is an inflammatory mediator that binds to the IL-1RI and triggers the inflammatory response. (Calabrese,2002; Arend, 2002)

- **Dosage** For moderate to severe active RA patients the recommended dosage of anakinra is 100 mg/day subcutaneously.

- **Adverse events** Most common and frequently reported side effect is injection site reaction and lasts for 15 days to 1 month. Other frequent side effects may include bacterial infection such as cellulitis, bone and joint infections, rather than unusual, opportunistic, fungal or viral infections. Serious infections may develop such as pneumonia or infections of the skin. (Fleischmann *et al.*, 2006; Mertens & Singh, 2009)

- **Clinical efficacy** In a study, 1,207 patients received 100 mg of anakinra in addition to DMARD (MTX, sulphasalazine or hydroxychloroquine) for up to 36 weeks (Le Loet *et al.*, 2008). Relevant improvement in the HAQ (Health Assessment Questionnaire) was seen in 51 %, with a DAS28 (Disease Activity Score- 28) amelioration of 1.5 at the end, without significant differences between the three DMARD patient groups. An assessment of using anakinra in RA involving 2,846 patients, of whom 781 and 2,065 were randomized to placebo and anakinra, respectively, concluded that anakinra demonstrated relative safety and modest efficacy in RA, although data for the long-term use are still being collected (Mertens & Singh, 2009).

Several biologics are already approved for the treatment of RA; however, no data are available/ published on any large study on head-to-head clinical trials to support using one agent over another. Nowadays, RA has an expanded range of available therapies and these provide a greater chance of controlling this disease. It is too early to say which molecule will be the most relevant target to hit for RA treatment. Early diagnosis of RA combined with early start of an appropriate treatment regimen is acknowledged as an important factor in improving clinical outcomes in patients with RA. Unfortunately, early diagnosis has been challenging because of the non-specific signs and symptoms associated with many polyarthropathies. However, with the advent of biologic drugs new imaging tools should be developed for selecting patients that may respond to one or other biological therapy.

3   Biosimilars and Intended Copies

Biologics, because of their complex structures, are variable and can never be duplicated, unlike small molecule drugs (generics) that are chemically synthesized (Zuñiga & Calvo, 2010). As the patents of biologics are expected to expire within the next few years, an opportunity has arose for the "biosimilars" to be marketed. A biosimilar is a biologic medicine that is similar but not the same to an already registered innovator biologic in terms of quality safety and efficacy. These molecules are also called as follow-on biologic (USA); subsequent entry biologic (Canada); similar biotherapeutic product (WHO) (Dranitsaris *et al.*, 2011).

Because the biosimilar manufacturers have no access to the production data of patented biologics, it is not possible to replicate the innovator. Variations in glycosylation, purification, formulation and storage may alter its safety, immunogenicity and efficacy profiles (Dorner *et al.*, 2013). Currently, several products labelled as "biosimilars" are approved for treatment of RA in a number of countries that, at the time of approval, did not have stringent regulatory processes in place to ensure comparability as defined by EMA (European Medical Agencies) and FDA. While these products apparently meet local regulatory requirements, they should be called "intended copies" (Dorner *et al.*,

2013). Thus any copy version of a biologic not developed and assessed in accordance with a strictly comparative development program should not be termed biosimilar (Weise *et al.*, 2011). Table 2 shows the intended copies of an Innovator biologic available in different parts of the world.

Biologics	Manufacturer	Intended Copy	Country
Rituximab	Dr. Reddy's Laboratories (India)	Reditux	Bolivia, Chile, Peru, India
Rituximab	Probiomed (Mexico)	Kikuzubam	Bolivia, Chile, Peru and Mexico
Etanercept	Shanghai CP Goujian Pharmaceutical Co (China)	Etanar	Colombia
Etanercept	Shanghai CP Goujian Pharmaceutical Co (China)	Yisaipu, Etacept	China and India

Table 2: Intended copies* of available biologics (Dorner *et al.*, 2013). * - Not as per EMA and FDA standards for biosimilars at time of approval

Though biosimilars may improve access to expensive biologics, their clinical benefit is still a question mark (Dorner *et al.*, 2013). While efficacy issues have been documented (Misra, 2012), the primary safety concern for biosimilar agents is their potential immunogenicity (Kessler *et al.*, 2006). Immune reactions like allergy, serum sickness, anaphylaxis as well as reduced or enhanced drug efficacy can occur (Schellekens, 2003). Quality (Misra, 2012) and interchangability (Sensabaugh, 2011) issues also need to be addressed. Practically, substitution of the innovator with a biosimilar can have clinical consequences as patients could respond differently to the two products. Thus, certain regulators like the EMA and the authorities in France, Germany, Greece, Italy, Slovenia, Spain, Sweden and UK do not permit substitution or interchangeability. Storage is a critical issue with biopharmaceuticals, particularly for when used and stored in conditions where temperature control could be a problem (Seshiah *et al.*, 2013). The same holds true for biosimilars (De Groot & Scott, 2007).

Because biosimilars are quite recent, clinicians should be aware of issues that have cropped up during their development and approval (Sekhon & Saluja, 2011). The use of biosimilars is essentially a change in clinical management (Combe *et al.*, 2005). They should be looked at more cautiously than generics. In addition, pharmacovigilance will be the need of the hour to track down any safety and efficacy problems with biosimilars. However, the wind of change is blowing in rheumatology. Rheumatologists are slowly getting exposed to "biosimilars". The role of biosimilars in the management of rheumatoid arthritis, however, will be based on the confidence gained by the treating rheumatologist. Rheumatologists will, sooner or later, be utilizing a wide range of alternative options to many patented originator biologics. It is likely that the implementation of biosimilars in the management of different rheumatic diseases will change the treatment algorithms we currently use, and this will be mainly based on the cost saved. Only hands-on experience will prove if many current beliefs will hold true (Noaiseh & Moreland, 2013). It is hoped that biosimilars will help improve patient access to expensive biologics. The success of an individual biosimilar will ultimately depend on the clinical data generated to support the product. However, it is important that clinicians distinguish between biological "intended copies" and biosimilars. Proper regulatory protocols need to be followed for getting a biosimilar approval. Issues regarding the safety, efficacy and similarity of biosimilars as compared to the innovator biologics have raised potential concerns regarding their use and should be addressed before giving them approval. Also, intended copies which do not comply to the regulatory standards for biosimilars have gained access in some countries which may lead to hazardous consequences. Patient safety and interchangeability of biosimilars will depend on establishment of stringent regulatory processes that best manage the potential benefits and risks associated with this newer drug category.

4   Clinical Considerations for Biological Therapy in RA

In the therapy for RA, the goal is to achieve and maintain remission or to minimize the disease activity. This may be possible by treating the patient to target, and maintaining tight disease-control. Regular monitoring of the disease activity, at 3 monthly intervals, is essential to evaluate the appropriateness of therapeutic approach. Early initiation of DMARDs facilitates the retardation of disease progression, and induction of more remissions. Synthetic DMARDs like methotrexate remain the agents of choice for initiation of therapy. Evidence suports the possibility of good initial control with biological agents, when used as first-line therapy. Improved initial control is also possible when biological agents are combined with synthetic DMARDs; however, the long-term sustenance of such benefit is not proven. In fact, this approach is considered to result in over-treatment, in a significant proportion of patients (van Vollenhoven, 2009). In early RA of < 6 months duration, the American College of Rheumatology (ACR) recommends the use of anti-TNF agents as first-line therapy, when the disease activity is high and prognosis is poor (ACR, 2012). In this scenario, the anti-TNF agents may be used with or without methotrexate; however, infliximab must always be used in combination with methotrexate. In established RA of ≥ 6 months' duration, the disease activity should be monitored every 3 months, to assess the influence of treatment. Inadequate control with synthetic DMARDs (monotherapy or combination therapy) should prompt the initiation of biological therapy.

4.1   Considerations for Initiating a Biological Therapy

Screening for latent tuberculosis infection, is suggested for all patients of RA (ACR, 2012). Screening may be carried out with Tuberculin Skin Test (TST) or Interferon Gamma Release Assays (IGRAs). IGRAs may be preferred over TST, as TST may give false-positive results in presence of BCG vaccination. In immunocompromized patients, screening tests may be falsely negative, and may be repeated after an interval of 1 to 3 weeks. Positive screening test result may prompt further assessment for active tuberculosis, with chest X-ray and sputum examination. In presence of latent tuberculosis, biological therapy may be considered after 1 month of anti-tuberculosis treatment, whereas in active tuberculosis, biological therapy may be considered only after completing the course of anti-tuberculosis therapy. When the risk of exposure to tuberculosis is present, periodic screening for tuberculosis infection may be considered, while continuing the biological therapy.

In patients with comorbidities like Hepatitis B or C, malignancy or congestive heart failure (CHF), the ACR has made special recommendations (ACR, 2012). For patients with hepatitis C, the use of etanercept is recommended. For patients with hepatitis B infection, the choice of biological agent is not conclusive. Biological therapy is not recommended if chronic hepatitis B is untreated, or even in treated cases, if the Child Pugh ranking is class B or higher. For patients with CHF with NYHA class III or IV, or when ejection fraction < 50%, therapy with anti-TNF agents is not recommended. In patients with previously treated solid cancers, skin cancers or lymphoproliferative cancers, rituximab may be used. If 5 years have elapsed after treatment for solid cancers or non-melanoma skin cancers, any biological agent may be considered.

4.2   Factors that Influence the Decision of Switching

In the biological therapy for RA, primary treatment failure following initiation, or secondary treatment failure after an initial response, are commonly encountered. For such cases, switching between biological agents is a reasonable option. The ACR recommends switching to different biological agents, in cases of observed loss or lack of benefit with the initial agents, or adverse reactions to the initial agents (ACR, 2012).

Safety profile of biological agents is an important consideration, and appearance of adverse effects is a valid reason to consider switching. TNF receptor fusion protein is known to be associated with lesser risk of reactivation tuberculosis, relative to anti-TNF monoclonal antibodies. Infusion reactions occurring with infliximab are common reasons for discontinuation and switching. In case of a serious adverse reaction developing to an anti-TNF agent, switching to a non-TNF agent must be considered. For serious or non-serious reactions developing to a non-TNF agent, switching to another non-TNF agent or to an anti-TNF agent may be considered.

Within the anti-TNF options, switching can result in improved outcomes owing to the different biological structures, affinities and half-lives. Appearance of neutralizing antibodies, against the therapeutic monoclonal antibodies, frequently results in loss of efficacy, over a period of time. This is a common reason to consider a switch to another biological agent, like a receptor fusion protein. Generally, such antibodies that develop against the fusion proteins are non-neutralizing, whereas those developing against the monoclonal antibodies possess the capacity of neutralization.

Primary treatment failure with any biological agent may indicate the active existence of different pathological mechanism(s). In such cases, it is prudent to switch to a biological agent, which acts on a different pathological target.

4.3   Achieving Remission and Tapering of TNF Therapy?

Sustained remission is the ideal goal of therapy in RA. The definitions of remission of RA for clinical practice, evolved by the ACR/EULAR task-force, are described in the Figure 1 (Zhang, *et al.*, 2012). Evidence to address the considerations of tapering DMARDs is not conclusive. Persistent remission for at least 12 months may be observed, for any considerations of therapeutic adjustments.

---

a)   **Boolean-based definition**

At any time point, patient must satisfy all of the following:

- Tender joint count (28) ≤ 1

- Swollen joint count (28) ≤ 1

- Patient global assessment ≤ 1 (on a 0 – 10 scale)

b)   **Index-based definition**

Clinical Disease Activity Index (CDAI) score of ≤ 2.8.

CDAI comprises of tender-28 joint count, swollen-28 joint count, patient global disease activity and evaluator's global disease activity.

Figure 1: Definition of Remission for Clinical Practice in RA (Zhang, et al., 2012). Definitions adapted from the ACR/EULAR definitions of remission in rheumatoid arthritis (Zhang *et al.*, 2012).

5   Lessons from the Biologics Registries

Clinical trials of TNF inhibitors (TNFi) have several limitations such as relatively fewer number of patients, limited exposure; exclusion of patients with co-morbidities; etc. Meta-analyses of Randomised controlled trials (RCT) have highlighted the "short term" safety profile of biologic therapies approved for RA. Since some of the adverse effects of interest are rare but severe, and occur during long-term use of biologics, we need to also look at non-randomized observational/registry studies to fully address the safety issues of biologic therapy for RA (Rawlins & De Testimonio, 2008) Also in the absence of head to head trials; questions regarding treatment comparisons may not be adequately answered by RCTs. (Rawlins & De Testimonio, 2008; Silman *et al.*, 2000; Zink *et al.*, 2009). Information from different national registries provides real-life, long-term data in patients with co-morbidities relevant to safety, efficacy and long-term outcomes (Zink *et al.*, 2009). Registries provide feedback on the management of rheumatic conditions in real life that can inform clinical decision making (Zink *et al.*, 2009). The growing importance of the registries is underlined by the fact that regulatory agencies, as well as the pharmaceutical industry, have identified the registries as useful post-marketing drug surveillance tools (Rawlins & De Testimonio, 2008). Long-term observational studies should be seen as complementary to RCTs and not as inferior data sources (Silman *et al.*, 2000; Zink *et al.*, 2009). Agreeing on a standardized reporting system for serious adverse events, and the ongoing discussions on methodological issues, have ensured that the registries have improved quality of data that is reported to regulatory agencies (Silman *et al.*, 2000). Re ulatory authorities in certain parts of the world now require patients on new drugs to be included in existing registries. This means that although the biological registries began as an academic enterprise with voluntary support from different pharmaceutical companies, they have evolved into official pharmacovigilance tools (Silman *et al.*, 2000). Primarily, registries obtain data on the real-life clinical use of TNFi to investigate long-term safety and efficacy. Registries provide real life feedback on the management of RA that can inform clinical decision making. A major advantage of the registries over industry-driven observational post-marketing studies is that all registeries follow up with patients irrespective of whether they continue treatment with a specific drug (Rawlins & De Testimonio, 2008).

However, there may be challenges to methodology of registries. Channeling bias or confounding by indication are obvious limitations and may be because treatment guidelines in some countries that limit the prescription of TNF inhibitors to patients with severe disease, a bad prognosis or those who have failed to respond to DMARD therapy (Zink *et al.*, 2009). Methods for controlling these biases and adjusting for confounding must be applied at several stages of the research process: selection biases have an influence not only at the start of biological treatment but also at clinical decision time points regarding "switching" to alternative drugs (Zink *et al.*, 2009). Choosing an adequate control group is difficult – matching on many different criteria is important and statistical methods need to be used to minimize confounding by indication when the data are analyzed (Zink *et al.*, 2009). Table 3 highlights the registries set across the world.

5.1   Safety Results for Registry Studies

5.1.1   Infections

The CORRONA database showed that in RA patients, higher disease activity was associated with a higher probability of developing infections (Au *et al.*, 2011). Askling and colleagues showed that RA patients are at increased risk of hospitalisation due to infection but this risk decreases as time from initiation of TNFi treatment increases. Within the RA cohort studied, the overall response rate (RR) for TNF inhibitor-associated infection, adjusted for comorbidity and use of inpatient care, was increased by approximately 30% during the first year of treatment Importantly, however, beyond the first year of follow-up on first TNF inhibitor treatment, no significant increase in infection risk was noted. Rates of severe infections were similar across the biologic treatment groups (Askling *et al.*, 2007). Compared with the DMARD-treated cohort; data from BSRBR reported no increased risk of all-site serious infection for any of the 3 TNF inhibitor therapies. There were 8,973 patients included in the analysis: 7,664 in the anti-TNF cohort (3,596 etanercept, 2,878 infliximab, 1,190 adalimumab) and 1,354 in the comparison cohort

Country	Name of Registry	Started	Total TNFi Treated Patients (year)
Sweden (Askling *et al.*, 2006)	ARTIS (STURE, SSATG)	1999	7354 (2006)
UK (Mercer *et al.*, 2009)	BSRBR	2001	11,757 (2009)
Germany (Zink *et al.*, 2013)	RABBIT	2001	7000 (2009)
Spain (Gomez-Reino *et al.*, 2003; "Spanish registry", 2014)	BIOBADASER	2000	5493 (2009)
Norway (Kvien *et al.*, 2005)	NOR-DMARD	2000	4683 (2005)
Denmark (Hetland, 2005)	DANBIO	2000	3056 (2005)
Czech Rep ("Attra Clinical Register", 2014)	ATTRA	2002	1403 (2009)
Netherlands (Kievit *et al.*, 2007)	DREAM	2003	546 (2007)
Italy (Marchesoni *et al.*, 2009)	LORHEN	1999	1114 (2009)
Switzerland (Pan *et al.*, 2009)	SCQM	1997	2364* (2009)
Greece (Flouri *et al.*, 2009)	HRBT	2004	715 (2009)
Japan (Komano *et al.*, 2011)	REAL	2005	1144 (2010)
US (Kremer, 2005)	CORRONA	2002	8755 (2005)
France (Salliot *et al.*, 2007)	RATIO	1997	1571 (2004)

Table 3: Worldwide Established Registries.

(Dixon *et al.*, 2006). Galloway and colleagues compared the risk of serious infections between 11,798 patients treated with infliximab, adalimumab, or etanercept and 3598 synthetic DMARDs patients using data from 2001 to 2009 in the British Society for Rheumatology Biologics Register (BSRBR) and the data suggest that anti-TNF therapy is associated with a small but significant overall risk of serious infection (Galloway *et al.*, 2011). The Dutch Rheumatoid Arthritis Monitoring (DREAM) register of 2157 RA patients showed the risk of serious infection in RA patients treated with either adalimumab or infliximab was similar (unadjusted hazard ratio of 3.31 and 4.13, respectively) (van Dartel *et al.*, 2011). However, risk of serious infection in RA patients treated with etanercept was significantly lower (unadjusted hazard ratio of 2.13) (van Dartel *et al.*, 2011). Even in the RATIO registry Patients on etanercept had lower rates of opportunistic infections vs. infliximab or adalimumab. (Salmon-Ceron *et al.*, 2011)

Tuberculosis (TB)
The data from the BSRBR registry showed that the rate of TB in patients with RA treated with anti-TNF therapy was three to fourfold higher in patients receiving infliximab or adalimumab than in those receiving etanercept (Dixon *et al.*, 2010). Similarly the French Research Axed on Tolerance of Biotherapies (RATIO) registry showed that the risk of TB is higher for patients receiving anti-TNF mAb therapy than for those receiving soluble TNF receptor therapy. The increased risk with early anti-TNF treatment and the ab-

sence of correct chemoprophylactic treatment favor the reactivation of latent TB (Tubach *et al.*, 2009).

Serious Viral Infections

While the RABBIT registry showed that the incidence of Herpes zoster increased in rheumatoid patients treated with infliximab or adalimumab but not etanercept (Strangeld *et al.*, 2009). No significant association with herpes zoster was found for etanercept use (HR, 1.36 [95% CI: 0.73-2.55]) (Strangeld *et al.*, 2009); the BSRBR registry showed that Varicella Zoster Virus (VZV) infections are increased in Patients with Rheumatoid Arthritis (RA) Treated with Anti-TNF Therapy (Galloway *et al.*, 2010). A similar pattern of risk was seen for each anti-TNF therapy with no statistical difference between etanercept and the monoclonal antibodies (Galloway *et al.*, 2010). Thus reactivation of herpes zoster is the most common viral problem associated with TNFi treatment. Data from BIOBADASER and BRSBR show very low rates of Listeria infection in TNFi treated rheumatoid patients (Pena *et al.*, 2008). Data from RATIO and BSRBR show very low rates of Legionella infection in TNFi treated patients (Tubach *et al.*, 2006).

5.1.2   Malignancies

According to ARTIS Registry data, RA patients in general have a marginally increased risk of solid cancers. The risk of cancer in RA patients varied by cancer site, with non-melanoma skin cancer at the highest increased risk (70%), and smoke-related cancers at the next highest (20-50%). However, RA patients have a decreased risk of both breast and colorectal cancers (20% and 25%, respectively) (Askling *et al*, 2005). However, data from Swedish and US registries and observational meta analyses show no overall increased risk of new cancers has been associated with TNFi treatment (Askling *et al.*, 2005; Wolfe & Michaud 2007). Observational meta analysis data indicate patients treated with TNFi have a significantly increased risk of both non melanoma skin cancer and melanoma (Wolfe & Michaud 2007). Risk of lymphoma is elevated in RA, particularly in patients with more severe disease (Greenberg *et al.*, 2011). Generally, TNFi are not associated with any major further increase in the already elevated lymphoma occurrence in RA (Baeklund *et al.*, 2006).

5.1.3   Cardiovascular Risk

TNFi use is associated with reduced risk of cardiovascular events in RA patients (Greenberg *et al.*, 2011; Askling & Dixon, 2011). In the CORRONA registry cohort, anti-TNF use resulted in a reduction in myocardial infarction, Transient ischaemic attacks (TIA)/stroke, cardiovascular-related death, and composite cardiovascular events compared to DMARD and Methotrexate treated patients (Greenberg *et al.*, 2011; Askling & Dixon, 2011). After adjusting (for age, gender, smoking status, diabetes, hypertension, dyslipidemia, previous Myocardial Infarction (MI) or stroke and modified health assessment questionnaire score, aspirin use, naproxen use, non-selective non-steroidal anti-inflammatory drug use, and cyclooxygenase-2 inhibitor use.); TNF antagonist use was associated with a reduced risk of the primary composite cardiovascular endpoint compared with non-biological DMARD use. However, methotrexate was not associated with a reduced risk (Greenberg *et al.*, 2011; Askling & Dixon, 2011). There have been postmarketing reports of worsening of congestive heart failure (CHF), with and without identifiable precipitating factors, in patients taking soluble TNF receptor (Immunex Corporation, 2013) There have been rare reports of new onset CHF, including CHF in patients without known preexisting cardiovascular disease. Physicians should exercise caution when using soluble TNF receptor in patients who also have heart failure, and monitor patients carefully (Immunex Corporation, 2013).

5.1.4   Demyelinating Disease Risk

All confirmed cases of demyelinating disease, optic neuritis, and multiple sclerosis (MS) in patients with rheumatic diseases treated with TNF- *a* antagonists were reviewed from 3 different sources: (1) the Spanish Registry of biological therapies in rheumatic diseases (BIOBADASER); (2) the Spanish Pharmacovigilance Database of Adverse Drug Reactions (FEDRA); and (3) a systematic review (PubMed, EMBASE, and the Cochrane Library). However, it is not clear whether TNF antagonists increase the incidence of demyelinating diseases in patients with rheumatic diseases. It is estimated that the rate of demyelinating diseases in patients with rheumatic diseases treated with TNF antagonists does not clearly differ from the expected rate in the population (Cruz Fernandez-Espatero *et al.*, 2011)

5.2   Discontinuation Rates of Biologic Therapy

Marchesoni *et al.* used data from the Lombardy Rheumatology Network (LOHREN) registry to evaluate drug survival in 1064 patients treated with either infliximab, adalimumab, or etanercept. Data showed that long-term survival of etanercept was better than that of both infliximab and adalimumab. The risk of discontinuing infliximab was mainly due to primary or secondary loss of efficacy, whereas the risk of discontinuing adalimumab was mainly due to adverse events (Marchesoni *et al.*, 2009). Markenson *et al.* performed a retrospective analysis of the data from the RADIUS registry , a 5-year observational registry of patients with RA, to determine time to first- and second-course discontinuation of etanercept, infliximab, and adalimumab. This analysis included 2418 patients. Discontinuations due to adverse events were significantly lower ($P = 0.0006$) for etanercept than for infliximab (etanercept, 14%; infliximab, 22%; adalimumab, 17%) (Markenson *et al.*, 2011). Similarly, Hong Kong registry data showed that drug retention is higher in patients treated with etanercept compared to those treated with infliximab. Patients treated with infliximab had a lower cumulative probability of drug retention due to lack of efficacy or due to adverse events compared with patients treated with etanercept (Mok, 2011).

5.2.1   Drug Survival

In the DANBIO Registry: drug survival; among etanercept, adalimumab, infliximab treated-patients, infliximab had the lowest drug survival. This trend was observed at 24, 48, 72, and 96 month follow-ups (Hetland *et al.*, 2010). Similarly in the GISEA Registry; at 4 years etanercept survival was significantly higher than infliximab or adalimumab survival ($P < 0.0001$). At this time-point, 51.4% of etanercept -treated patients were remaining on therapy, 36.4% of adalimumab-treated patients were remaining on therapy, and 37.6% of infliximab-treated patients were remaining on therapy (Iannone *et al.*, 2011). ATTRA registry data demonstrated that Ankylosing Spondylitis patients were more adherent to anti-TNF therapy than RA patients (Pavelka *et al.*, 2009).

While registries provide valuable real life treatment information their observational nature, lack of controls and randomization require complex analysis to avoid confounding factors (Kievit *et al.*, 2007; Markenson *et al.*, 2011; Mok, 2011).

6   Future Perspectives in the Treatment of RA

Biologics go a long way towards meeting the needs of many RA patients. However there are patients who can fail biologics. Cost is an overriding factor in the development of newer molecules for targeted therapy of RA (Van Vallenhoven, 2010). Clinicians look for are therapies that are targeted; affordable and with an improved safety profile.

There are a large number of possible targets for modulating the immune response. Hence the current developments include biologics with different specific targets. Many novel biologics are undergoing development in RA e.g. newer IL-1 inhibitors, B-cell depleting agents osrelizumba, ofotumumab, TRUo15, targeting cytokines in B-cell maturation Bly5 inhibitor, AORUK inhibitor, briobacept, atitacept (Kukar *et al.*, 2009).

Another entirely new approach to treat RA is related to the development of small molecule compounds with similar targeted action and therapeutic efficacies (Van Vallenhoven, 2010). These include JAK-3 inhibitors (tofacitinib), Syk inhibitors (tamatinib, fosdium, lymphotoxin*B*, and LIGHT pathway inhibitors (baminercept), p38 MAP inhibitors (VX 702, SB-6811323) (Kukar *et al.*, 2009). Of these tofacitinib is marketed in many countries across the world.

Small molecule derivatives that target signal pathways that subserve the cytokine effector pathways are also attracting attention. Other approaches include the inhibition of factors that promote angiogenesis and those that promote osteolcast activation (anti-RANKL [anti-receptor activator of nuclear factor-kB ligand]) and modulate adipocytokines.

7   Conclusions

Biological therapy has undoubtedly been a subject of immense clinical interest, over the past few years. The resultant developments have engendered various perspectives for consideration, towards optimizing the therapeutic approach to RA. As a routine practice, biological agents are initiated following inadequate response to synthetic DMARDs. However, supportive evidence does prompt considerations for early use of biological agents, in the course of disease. An increase in the variety of available biologics has broadened the choice, propelling the approach towards personalized medicine. Long-term observations with biological therapies are now available, to help address some essential questions. Facilitated by the advent of more affordable biosimilar agents, improving the therapeutic access is now a real possibility.

References

AbbVie Inc (2014). Humira (adalimumab): Prescribing information. Retrieved from http://www.rxabbvie.com/pdf/humira.pdf accessed on 30th September 2014.

American College of Rheumatology. (2012). 2012 Update of the 2008 American College of Rheumatology recommendations for the use of disease-modifying antirheumatic drugs and biologic agents in the treatment of rheumatoid arthritis. Arthritis care & research, 64(5), 625–639.

Anderson, P. J. (2005, April). Tumor necrosis factor inhibitors: clinical implications of their different immunogenicity profiles. In Seminars in arthritis and rheumatism (Vol. 34, No. 5, pp. 19–22). WB Saunders.

Arend, W. P. (2002). The mode of action of cytokine inhibitors. The Journal of Rheumatology, 65, 16–21.

Askling, J., & Dixon, W. (2011). Influence of biological agents on cardiovascular disease in rheumatoid arthritis. Annals of the rheumatic diseases, 70(4), 561–562.

Askling, J., Fored, C. M., Baecklund, E., Brandt, L., Backlin, C., Ekbom, A., ... & Feltelius, N. (2005). Haematopoietic malignancies in rheumatoid arthritis: lymphoma risk and characteristics after exposure to tumour necrosis factor antagonists. Annals of the rheumatic diseases, 64(10), 1414–1420.

Askling, J., Fored, C. M., Brandt, L., Baecklund, E., Bertilsson, L., Feltelius, N., ... & Klareskog, L. (2007). Time-dependent increase in risk of hospitalisation with infection among Swedish RA patients treated with TNF antagonists. Annals of the rheumatic diseases, 66(10), 1339–1344.

Askling, J., Fored, C. M., Geborek, P., Jacobsson, L. T., van Vollenhoven, R., Feltelius, N., ... & Klareskog, L. (2006). Swedish registers to examine drug safety and clinical issues in RA. Annals of the rheumatic diseases, 65(6), 707–712.

Askling, J., van Vollenhoven, R. F., Granath, F., Raaschou, P., Fored, C. M., Baecklund, E., ... & Klareskog, L. (2009). Cancer risk in patients with rheumatoid arthritis treated with anti–tumor necrosis factor α therapies: Does the risk change with the time since start of treatment?. Arthritis & Rheumatism,60(11), 3180–3189.

Attra Clinical Register. Available at: www.attra.registry.cz.; accessed on 30th September 2014

Au, K., Reed, G., Curtis, J. R., Kremer, J. M., Greenberg, J. D., Strand, V., & Furst, D. E. (2011). High disease activity is associated with an increased risk of infection in patients with rheumatoid arthritis. Annals of the rheumatic diseases.

Baecklund, E., Iliadou, A., Askling, J., Ekbom, A., Backlin, C., Granath, F., ... & Klareskog, L. (2006). Association of chronic inflammation, not its treatment, with increased lymphoma risk in rheumatoid arthritis. Arthritis & Rheumatism,54(3), 692–701.

Bain, B., & Brazil, M. (2003). Adalimumab. Nature Reviews Drug Discovery,2(9), 693–694.

Biogen Idec, Inc (2014). Rituxan (rituximab): Prescribing information. Retrieved from http://www.gene.com/download/pdf/rituxan_prescribing.pdf accessed on 30th September 2014.

Boonen, A., & Severens, J. L. (2011). The burden of illness of rheumatoid arthritis. Clinical rheumatology, 30(1), 3–8.

Breedveld, F. C., Weisman, M. H., Kavanaugh, A. F., Cohen, S. B., Pavelka, K., Vollenhoven, R. V., ... & Spencer-Green, G. T. (2006). The PREMIER study: a multicenter, randomized, double-blind clinical trial of combination therapy with adalimumab plus methotrexate versus methotrexate alone or adalimumab alone in patients with early, aggressive rheumatoid arthritis who had not had previous methotrexate treatment. Arthritis & Rheumatism, 54(1), 26–37.

Brennan, F. M., Chantry, D., Jackson, A. M., Maini, R. N., & Feldmann, M. (1989). Cytokine production in culture by cells isolated from the synovial membrane. Journal of autoimmunity, 2, 177–186.

Bristol-Myers Squibb, Company (2013). Orencia (abatacept): Prescribing information. Retrieved from http://packageinserts.bms.com/pi/pi_orencia.pdf accessed on 30th September 2014

Buchan, G., Barrett, K., Turner, M., Chantry, D., Maini, R. N., & Feldmann, M. (1988). Interleukin-1 and tumour necrosis factor mRNA expression in rheumatoid arthritis: prolonged production of IL-1 alpha. Clinical and experimental immunology, 73(3), 449.

Burmester, G. R., Mariette, X., Montecucco, C., Monteagudo-Sáez, I., Malaise, M., Tzioufas, A. G., ... & Kupper, H. (2007). Adalimumab alone and in combination with disease-modifying antirheumatic drugs for the treatment of rheumatoid arthritis in clinical practice: the Research in Active Rheumatoid Arthritis (ReAct) trial. Annals of the rheumatic diseases, 66(6), 732–739.

Calabrese, L. H. (2002). Molecular differences in anticytokine therapies. Clinical and experimental rheumatology, 21(2), 241–248.

Combe, C., Tredree, R. L., & Schellekens, H. (2005). Biosimilar epoetins: an analysis based on recently implemented European medicines evaluation agency guidelines on comparability of biopharmaceutical proteins. Pharmacotherapy: The Journal of Human Pharmacology and Drug Therapy,25(7), 954–962.

Cruz Fernández-Espartero, M., Pérez-Zafrilla, B., Naranjo, A., Esteban, C., Ortiz, A. M., Gómez-Reino, J. J., & Carmona, L. (2011, December). Demyelinating disease in patients treated with TNF antagonists in rheumatology: data from BIOBADASER, a *pharmacovigilance database, and a systematic review. In Seminars in arthritis and rheumatism (Vol. 41, No. 3, pp. 524–533). WB Saunders.*

De Groot, A. S., & Scott, D. W. (2007). *Immunogenicity of protein therapeutics. Trends in immunology, 28(11), 482–490.*

Dixon, W. G., Hyrich, K. L., Watson, K. D., Lunt, M., Galloway, J., Ustianowski, A., & Symmons, D. P. M. (2010). *Drug-specific risk of tuberculosis in patients with rheumatoid arthritis treated with anti-TNF therapy: results from the British Society for Rheumatology Biologics Register (BSRBR).Annals of the rheumatic diseases, 69(3), 522–528.*

Dixon, W. G., Watson, K., Lunt, M., Hyrich, K. L., Silman, A. J., & Symmons, D. P. (2006). *British Society for Rheumatology Biologics Register. Rates of serious infection, including site-specific and bacterial intracellular infection, in rheumatoid arthritis patients receiving anti-tumor necrosis factor therapy: results from the British Society for Rheumatology Biologics Register. Arthritis Rheum,54(8), 2368–2376.*

Dörner, T., Strand, V., Castañeda-Hernández, G., Ferraccioli, G., Isaacs, J. D., Kvien, T. K., ... & Burmester, G. R. (2013). *The role of biosimilars in the treatment of rheumatic diseases. Annals of the rheumatic diseases, 72(3), 322–328.*

Dranitsaris, G., Amir, E., & Dorward, K. (2011). *Biosimilars of biological drug therapies. Drugs, 71(12), 1527–1536.*

Edwards, J. C., Szczepański, L., Szechiński, J., Filipowicz-Sosnowska, A., Emery, P., Close, D. R., ... & Shaw, T. (2004). *Efficacy of B-cell–targeted therapy with rituximab in patients with rheumatoid arthritis. New England Journal of Medicine, 350(25), 2572–2581.*

Elliott MJ, Maini RN, Feldmann M, Long-Fox A, Charles P, Katsikis P, Brennan FM, Walker J, Bijl H, Ghrayeb J (1993) *Treatment of rheumatoid arthritis with chimeric monoclonal antibodies to tumor necrosis factor a. Arthritis Rheum 36:1681–1690*

Emery P, Fleischmann RM, Moreland LW, Hsia EC, Strusberg I, Durez P, et al (2009). *Golimumab, a new human anti-tumor necrosis factor-a monoclonal antibody, injected subcutaneously every four weeks in methotrexate-naïve patients with active rheumatoid arthritis. Arthritis Rheumatol, 60, 2272–83.*

Emery, P., Breedveld, F. C., Hall, S., Durez, P., Chang, D. J., Robertson, D., ... & Freundlich, B. (2008). *Comparison of methotrexate monotherapy with a combination of methotrexate and etanercept in active, early, moderate to severe rheumatoid arthritis (COMET): a randomised, double-blind, parallel treatment trial. The Lancet, 372(9636), 375–382.*

Emery, P., Kosinski, M., Li, T., Martin, M., Williams, G. R., Becker, J. C., ... & Russell, A. S. (2006). *Treatment of rheumatoid arthritis patients with abatacept and methotrexate significantly improved health-related quality of life. The Journal of rheumatology, 33(4), 681–689.*

Fan, P., & Leong, K. (2007). *The use of biological agents in the treatment of rheumatoid arthritis. Annals-Academy of Medicine Singapore, 36(2), 128.*

Feldmann M, Brennan FM, Maini RN (1996) *Role of cytokines in rheumatoid arthritis. Annu Rev Immunol 14:397–440*

Feldmann M, Maini RN (2001). Anti-TNF-a therapy of rheumatoid arthritis: what have we learned? Annu Rev Immunol, 19, 163–96.

Fleischmann, R. M., Tesser, J., Schiff, M. H., Schechtman, J., Burmester, G. R., Bennett, R., ... & Appleton, B. (2006). Safety of extended treatment with anakinra in patients with rheumatoid arthritis. Annals of the rheumatic diseases,65(8), 1006–1012.

Fleischmann, R., Vencovsky, J., van Vollenhoven, R. F., Borenstein, D., Box, J., Coteur, G., ... & Strand, V. (2009). Efficacy and safety of certolizumab pegol monotherapy every 4 weeks in patients with rheumatoid arthritis failing previous disease-modifying antirheumatic therapy: the FAST4WARD study. Annals of the rheumatic diseases, 68(6), 805–811.

Galloway, J. B., Hyrich, K. L., Mercer, L. K., Dixon, W. G., Fu, B., Ustianowski, A. P., ... & Symmons, D. P. (2011). Anti-TNF therapy is associated with an increased risk of serious infections in patients with rheumatoid arthritis especially in the first 6 months of treatment: updated results from the British Society for Rheumatology Biologics Register with special emphasis on risks in the elderly. Rheumatology, 50(1), 124–131.

Gardam MA, Keystone EC, Menzies R, Manners S, Skamene E, Long R, et al. (2003). Anti-tumor necrosis factor agents and tuberculosis risk: mechanisms of action and clinical management. Lancet Infect Dis, 3, 148–55.

Genovese, M. C., Bathon, J. M., Martin, R. W., Fleischmann, R. M., Tesser, J. R., Schiff, M. H., ... & Finck, B. K. (2002). Etanercept versus methotrexate in patients with early rheumatoid arthritis: two-year radiographic and clinical outcomes. Arthritis & Rheumatism, 46(6), 1443–1450.

Genovese, M. C., McKay, J. D., Nasonov, E. L., Mysler, E. F., da Silva, N. A., Alecock, E., ... & Gomez-Reino, J. J. (2008). Interleukin-6 receptor inhibition with tocilizumab reduces disease activity in rheumatoid arthritis with inadequate response to disease-modifying antirheumatic drugs: The tocilizumab in combination with traditional disease-modifying antirheumatic drug therapy study. Arthritis & Rheumatism, 58(10), 2968–2980.

Gómez-Reino, J. J., Carmona, L., Valverde, V. R., Mola, E. M., & Montero, M. D. (2003). Treatment of rheumatoid arthritis with tumor necrosis factor inhibitors may predispose to significant increase in tuberculosis risk: a multicenter active-surveillance report. Arthritis & Rheumatism, 48(8), 2122–2127.

Greenberg, J. D., Kremer, J. M., Curtis, J. R., Hochberg, M. C., Reed, G., Tsao, P., ... & Solomon, D. H. (2011). Tumour necrosis factor antagonist use and associated risk reduction of cardiovascular events among patients with rheumatoid arthritis. Annals of the rheumatic diseases, 70(4), 576–582.

Hetland, M. L. (2005). DANBIO: a nationwide registry of biological therapies in Denmark. Clinical and experimental rheumatology, 23(5), S205.

Hetland, M. L., Christensen, I. J., Tarp, U., Dreyer, L., Hansen, A., Hansen, I. T., ... & Østergaard, M. (2010). Direct comparison of treatment responses, remission rates, and drug adherence in patients with rheumatoid arthritis treated with adalimumab, etanercept, or infliximab: results from eight years of surveillance of clinical practice in the nationwide Danish Danbio registry. Arthritis & Rheumatism, 62(1), 22–32.

Hirohata S (2007). *Fully human anti TNF-alpha monoclonal antibodies (adalimumab, golimumab). Nippon Rinsho, 65, 1202–28.*

Iannone, F., Gremese, E., Atzeni, F., Biasi, D., Botsios, C., Cipriani, P., ... & Trotta, F. (2012). *Longterm retention of tumor necrosis factor-α inhibitor therapy in a large italian cohort of patients with rheumatoid arthritis from the GISEA registry: an appraisal of predictors. The Journal of rheumatology, 39(6), 1179–1184.*

Immunex Corporation (2013). *Enbrel (etanercept): Prescribing information. Retrieved from http://pi.amgen.com/united_states/enbrel/derm/enbrel_pi.pdf accessed on 30th September 2014*

Indian Guidelines for the management of rheumatoid arthritis (2002). *JAPI, 50, 1207–1218*

Janssen Biotech Inc (2013a). *Remicade (infliximab): Prescribing information. Retrieved: http://www.remicade.com/shared/product/remicade/prescribing-information.pdf accessed on 30th September, 2014*

Janssen Biotech, Inc (2013b). *Simponi (golimumab): Prescribing information. Retrieved from http://www.simponi.com/shared/product/simponi/prescribing-information.pdf accessed on 30th September 2014.*

Kessler, M., Goldsmith, D., & Schellekens, H. (2006). *Immunogenicity of biopharmaceuticals. Nephrology Dialysis Transplantation, 21(suppl 5), v9-v12.*

Keystone, E. C., Genovese, M. C., Klareskog, L., Hsia, E. C., Hall, S. T., Miranda, P. C., ... & Rahman, M. U. (2008a). *Golimumab, a human antibody to TNF-α given by monthly subcutaneous injections, in active rheumatoid arthritis despite methotrexate: The GO-FORWARD Study. Annals of the rheumatic diseases. 68(6), 789–96.*

Keystone, E.C., Heijde, D. V. D., Mason, D., Landewé, R., Vollenhoven, R. V., Combe, B., ... & Pavelka, K. (2008b). *Certolizumab pegol plus methotrexate is significantly more effective than placebo plus methotrexate in active rheumatoid arthritis: Findings of a fifty-two–week, phase III, multicenter, randomized, double-blind, placebo-controlled, parallel-group study. Arthritis & Rheumatism, 58(11), 3319–3329.*

Kievit, W., Fransen, J., Oerlemans, A. J. M., Kuper, H. H., Van Der Laar, M. A. F. J., de Rooij, D. J. R. A. M., ... & van Riel, P. L. C. M. (2007). *The efficacy of anti-TNF in rheumatoid arthritis, a comparison between randomised controlled trials and clinical practice. Annals of the rheumatic diseases, 66(11), 1473–1478*

Komano, Y., Tanaka, M., Nanki, T., Koike, R., Sakai, R., Kameda, H., ... & Migita, K. (2011). *Incidence and risk factors for serious infection in patients with rheumatoid arthritis treated with tumor necrosis factor inhibitors: a report from the Registry of Japanese Rheumatoid Arthritis Patients for Longterm Safety. The Journal of rheumatology, 38(7), 1258–1264.*

Kremer, J. (2005). *The CORRONA database. Annals of the rheumatic diseases, 64 (suppl 4), iv37–iv41.*

Kremer, J., Fleischmann, R., Brzezicki, J., Ambs, P., Alecock, E., Burgos-Vargas, R., & Halland, A. (2009). *Tocilizumab inhibits structural joint damage, improves physical function, and increases DAS28 remission rates in RA patients who respond inadequately to methotrexate:*

the LITHE study. Ann Rheum Dis, 68(Suppl 3), 122.s

Kukar, M., Petryna, O., & Efthimiou, P. (2009). Biological targets in the treatment of rheumatoid arthritis: a comprehensive review of current and in-development biological disease modifying anti-rheumatic drugs. Biologics: targets & therapy, 3, 443.

Kvien, T. K. (2004). Epidemiology and burden of illness of rheumatoid arthritis. Pharmacoeconomics, 22(1), 1–12.

Kvien, T. K., Heiberg, M. S., Lie, E., Kaufmann, C., Mikkelsen, K., Nordvag, B., & Rodevand, E. (2005). A Norwegian DMARD register: prescriptions of DMARDs and biological agents to patients with inflammatory rheumatic diseases. Clinical and experimental rheumatology, 23(5), S188

Le Loet, X., NORDSTRÖM, D., Rodriguez, M., Rubbert, A., Sarzi-Puttini, P., Wouters, J. M., ... & Appleton, B. (2008). Effect of anakinra on functional status in patients with active rheumatoid arthritis receiving concomitant therapy with traditional disease modifying antirheumatic drugs: evidence from the OMEGA Trial. The Journal of rheumatology, 35(8), 1538–1544.

Linsley, P. S., Wallace, P. M., Johnson, J., Gibson, M. G., Greene, J. L., Ledbetter, J. A., ... & Tepper, M. A. (1992). Immunosuppression in vivo by a soluble form of the CTLA-4 T cell activation molecule. Science, 257(5071), 792–795.

Lipsky PE, van der Heijde DM, St Clair EW, Furst DE, Breedveld FC, Kalden JR, Smolen JS, Weisman M, Emery P, Feldmann M, Harriman GR, Maini RN (2000) Infliximab and methotrexate in the treatment of rheumatoid arthritis. Anti-Tumor Necrosis Factor Trial in Rheumatoid Arthritis with Concomitant Therapy Study Group. N Engl J Med 343:1594–602

Lundkvist J, Kastang F, Kobelt G (2008) The burden of rheumatoid arthritis and access .Eur J Health Econ 8:S49–S60

Marchesoni, A., Zaccara, E., Gorla, R., Bazzani, C., Sarzi-Puttini, P., Atzeni, F., ... & Favalli, E. G. (2009). TNF-α Antagonist Survival Rate in a Cohort of Rheumatoid Arthritis Patients Observed under Conditions of Standard Clinical Practice. Annals of the New York Academy of Sciences, 1173(1), 837–846

Mariette, X., Matucci-Cerinic, M., Pavelka, K., Taylor, P., van Vollenhoven, R., Heatley, R., ... & Emery, P. (2011). Malignancies associated with tumour necrosis factor inhibitors in registries and prospective observational studies: a systematic review and meta-analysis. Annals of the rheumatic diseases, annrheumdis149419.

Markenson, J. A., Gibofsky, A., Palmer, W. R., Keystone, E. C., Schiff, M. H., Feng, J., & Baumgartner, S. W. (2011). Persistence with anti-tumor necrosis factor therapies in patients with rheumatoid arthritis: observations from the RADIUS registry. The Journal of rheumatology, jrheum-101142.

Mercer, L. K., Green, A. C., Galloway, J. B., Davies, R., Lunt, M., Dixon, W. G., ... & Hyrich, K. L. (2012). The influence of anti-TNF therapy upon incidence of keratinocyte skin cancer in patients with rheumatoid arthritis: longitudinal results from the British Society for

Rheumatology Biologics Register. Annals of the rheumatic diseases, 71(6), 869–874.

Mertens M, Singh JA (2009),
Anakinra for rheumatoid arthritis: systematic review. J Rheumatol 36: 1118–1125.

Misra, M. (2012). *Biosimilars: Current perspectives and future implications. Indian journal of pharmacology, 44(1), 12.*

Misra, R., Sharma, B. L., Gupta, R., Pandya, S., Agarwal, S., Agarwal, P., ... & Wangjam, K. (2008). *Indian Rheumatology Association consensus statement on the management of adults with rheumatoid arthritis. Indian Journal of Rheumatology, 3(3), S1–S16.*

Mok CC (2011). *Lessons from biologics registries: efficacy and drug survival in RA. Rheumatology News, 6, 8–9.*

Moreland, L., Bate, G., & Kirkpatrick, P. (2006). *Abatacept. Nature Reviews Drug Discovery, 5(3), 185–186.*

Nesbitt, A. M., & Henry, A. J. (2004, October). *High affinity and potency of the PEGylated Fab'fragment CDP870-A direct comparison with other anti-TNF agents. In American Journal of Gastroenterology (Vol. 99, No. 10, pp. S253–S253). Blackwell Publishing Inc.*

Noaiseh, G., & Moreland, L. (2013). *Current and future biosimilars: potential practical applications in rheumatology. Biosimilars, 3.*

Olszewski, A. J., & Grossbard, M. L. (2004). *Empowering targeted therapy: lessons from rituximab. Science Signaling, 2004(241), pe30.*

Pan, S. M. D., Dehler, S., Ciurea, A., Ziswiler, H. R., Gabay, C., & Finckh, A. (2009). *Comparison of drug retention rates and causes of drug discontinuation between anti–tumor necrosis factor agents in rheumatoid arthritis. Arthritis Care & Research, 61(5), 560–568.*

Pavelka, K., Forejtova, S., Stolfa, J., Chroust, K., Buresova, L., Mann, H., & Vencovský, J. (2009). *Anti-TNF therapy of ankylosing spondylitis in clinical practice. Results from the Czech national registry ATTRA. Clin Exp Rheumatol,27(6), 958–963.*

Peña-Sagredo, J. L., Hernández, M. V., Fernandez-Llanio, N., Giménez-Ubeda, E., Munoz-Fernandez, S., Ortiz, A., ... & Fariñas, M. C. (2008). *Listeria monocytogenes infection in patients with rheumatic diseases on TNF-alpha antagonist therapy: the Spanish Study Group experience. Clinical & Experimental Rheumatology, 26(5), 854.*

Rau, R. (2002). *Adalimumab (a fully human anti-tumour necrosis factor α monoclonal antibody) in the treatment of active rheumatoid arthritis: the initial results of five trials. Annals of the rheumatic diseases, 61(suppl 2), ii70–ii73.*

Rawlins, M. (2008). *De Testimonio: Harveian Oration Delivered to the Royal College of Physicians. Lancet, 372, 2152–2161.*

Reiser, H., & Stadecker, M. J. (1996). *Costimulatory B7 molecules in the pathogenesis of infectious and autoimmune diseases. New England Journal of Medicine, 335(18), 1369–1377.*

Salliot, C., Gossec, L., Ruyssen-Witrand, A., Luc, M., Duclos, M., Guignard, S., & Dougados, M. (2007). *Infections during tumour necrosis factor-α blocker therapy for rheumatic diseases in daily practice: a systematic retrospective study of 709 patients. Rheumatology, 46(2), 327–334.*

Salmon-Céron, D., Tubach, F., Lortholary, O., Chosidow, O., Bretagne, S., Nicolas, N., ... & Mariette, X. (2011). *Drug-specific risk of non-tuberculosis opportunistic infections in patients receiving anti-TNF therapy reported to the 3-year prospective French RATIO registry. Annals of the rheumatic diseases,70(4), 616–623.*

Sato, K., Tsuchiya, M., Saldanha, J., Koishihara, Y., Ohsugi, Y., Kishimoto, T., & Bendig, M. M. (1993). *Reshaping a human antibody to inhibit the interleukin 6-dependent tumor cell growth. Cancer Research, 53(4), 851–856.*

Scallon BJ, Moore MA, Trinh H, Knight DM, Ghrayeb J (1995) *Chimeric anti-TNF a monoclonal antibody cA2 binds recombinant transmembrane TNFa and activates immune effector functions. Cytokine 7:251–259*

Schellekens, H (2003) *Immunogenicity of biopharmaceuticals: why proteins should be treated with respect Eur J Hosp Pharm. 112, 88–91.*

Sekhon, B. S., & Saluja, V. (2011). *Biosimilars: an overview. Biosimilars, 1(1), 1–11.*

Sensabaugh, S. M. (2011). *Requirements for Biosimilars and Interchangeable Biological Drugs in the United States—in Plain Language. Drug Information Journal, 45(2), 155–162.*

Seshiah V, Das AK, Sethi BK, Moses CRA, Kumar A, Viswanathan V, et al (2013). *Biopharmaceuticals and Biosimilars: A Consensus Statement. In: Medicine update, 5, 237–41. Available at: http://www.apiindia.org/medicine_update_2013/chap52.pdf. Accessed on 30th September 2014*

Sidiropoulos, P., Flouri, I., Drosos, A., Boki, K., Papadopoulos, I., Skopouli, F., ... & Boumpas, D. (2009). *Long-term follow-up of RA patients of the Hellenic Biologics Registry: comparison of first versus second anti-TNF-alpha therapy. Clinical and Experimental Rheumatology, 27(5), 708–708.*

Silman A, Klareskog L, Breedveld Fm Bresnihan B, Maini Rm van Riel P.I.E.T. & Symmonds, D (2000). *Proposal to establish a register for the long term surveillance of adverse events in patients with rheumatic diseases e posed to biological agents: the EULAR Surveillance Register for Biological Compounds. Annals of the rheumatic diseases, 59(6), 419–420.*

Smolen, J. S., Han, C., Bala, M., Maini, R. N., Kalden, J. R., Van der Heijde, D., ... & Lipsky, P. E. (2005). *Evidence of radiographic benefit of treatment with infliximab plus methotrexate in rheumatoid arthritis patients who had no clinical improvement: a detailed subanalysis of data from the Anti–Tumor Necrosis Factor Trial in Rheumatoid Arthritis with Concomitant Therapy study. Arthritis & Rheumatism, 52(4), 1020–1030.*

Smolen, J. S., Beaulieu, A., Rubbert-Roth, A., Ramos-Remus, C., Rovensky, J., Alecock, E., ... & Alten, R. (2008). *Effect of interleukin-6 receptor inhibition with tocilizumab in patients with rheumatoid arthritis (OPTION study): a double-blind, placebo-controlled, randomised trial. The Lancet, 371(9617), 987–997.*

Smolen, J. S., Landewé, R. B., Mease, P. H. I. L. I. P., Brzezicki, J., Mason, D., Luijtens, K., ... & Van Der Heijde, D. (2009a). *Efficacy and safety of certolizumab pegol plus methotrexate in active rheumatoid arthritis: the RAPID 2 study. A randomised controlled trial. Annals of the rheumatic diseases, 68(6), 797–804.*

Smolen, J. S., Kay, J., Doyle, M. K., Landewé, R., Matteson, E. L., Wollenhaupt, J., ... & Rahman, M. U. (2009b). Golimumab in patients with active rheumatoid arthritis after treatment with tumour necrosis factor α inhibitors (GO-AFTER study): a multicentre, randomised, double-blind, placebo-controlled, phase III trial. The Lancet, 374(9685), 210–221.

Spanish registry of adverse events of biological therapies in rheumatic diseases (Phase II). BIOBADASER November 2009 Report. Available at: http://biobadaser.ser. es/biobadaser/eng/docs/report_web_nov09_eng.pdf; accessed on 30th September 2014

St Clair, E. W., van der Heijde, D. M., Smolen, J. S., Maini, R. N., Bathon, J. M., ... & Baker, D. (2004). Combination of infliximab and methotrexate therapy for early rheumatoid arthritis: a randomized, controlled trial. Arthritis & Rheumatism, 50(11), 3432–3443.

Stern, M., & Herrmann, R. (2005). Overview of monoclonal antibodies in cancer therapy: present and promise. Critical reviews in oncology/hematology, 54(1), 11–29.

Strangfeld, A., Listing, J., Herzer, P., Liebhaber, A., Rockwitz, K., Richter, C., & Zink, A. (2009). Risk of herpes zoster in patients with rheumatoid arthritis treated with anti–TNF-α agents. Jama, 301(7), 737–744.

Tubach, F., Ravaud, P., Salmon-Ceron, D., Petitpain, N., Brocq, O., Grados, F., ... & Lortholary, O. (2006). Emergence of Legionella pneumophila Pneumonia in Patients Receiving Tumor Necrosis Factor–α Antagonists.Clinical Infectious Diseases, 43(10), e95–e100.

Tubach, F., Salmon, D., Ravaud, P., Allanore, Y., Goupille, P., Bréban, M., ... & Mariette, X. (2009). Risk of tuberculosis is higher with anti–tumor necrosis factor monoclonal antibody therapy than with soluble tumor necrosis factor receptor therapy: The three-year prospective french research axed on tolerance of biotherapies registry. Arthritis & Rheumatism, 60(7), 1884–1894.

Van Dartel, S., Fransen, J., & Kievit, W. (2011). The difference between adalimumab, infliximab and etanercept on the risk of serious infections in patients with rheumatoid arthritis: results from the DREAM registry. Ann Rheum Dis, 70 (Suppl 3), 417.

van der Heijde, D., Klareskog, L., Rodriguez-Valverde, V., Codreanu, C., Bolosiu, H., Melo-Gomes, J., ... & Fatenejad, S. (2006). Comparison of etanercept and methotrexate, alone and combined, in the treatment of rheumatoid arthritis: two-year clinical and radiographic results from the TEMPO study, a double-blind, randomized trial. Arthritis & Rheumatism, 54(4), 1063–1074.

van Vollenhoven, R. F. (2009). Treatment of rheumatoid arthritis: state of the art 2009. Nature Reviews Rheumatology, 5(10), 531–541.

van Vollenhoven, R. F. (2010). New and future agents in the treatment of rheumatoid arthritis. Discovery medicine, 9(47), 319–327

Weinblatt, M. E., Keystone, E. C., Furst, D. E., Kavanaugh, A. F., Chartash, E. K., & Segurado, O. G. (2006). Long term efficacy and safety of adalimumab plus methotrexate in patients with rheumatoid arthritis: ARMADA 4 year extended study. Annals of the rheumatic diseases, 65(6), 753–759.

Weinblatt, M. E., Keystone, E. C., Furst, D. E., Moreland, L. W., Weisman, M. H., Birbara, C. A., ... & Chartash, E. K. (2003). Adalimumab, a fully human anti–tumor necrosis factor α monoclonal antibody, for the treatment of rheumatoid arthritis in patients taking concomitant methotrexate: the ARMADA trial. Arthritis & Rheumatism, 48(1), 35–45.

Weinblatt, M., Combe, B., Covucci, A., Aranda, R., Becker, J. C., & Keystone, E. (2006). Safety of the selective costimulation modulator abatacept in rheumatoid arthritis patients receiving background biologic and nonbiologic disease-modifying antirheumatic drugs: A one-year randomized, placebo-controlled study. Arthritis & Rheumatism, 54(9), 2807–2816.

Weise, M., Bielsky, M. C., De Smet, K., Ehmann, F., Ekman, N., Narayanan, G., ... & Schneider, C. K. (2011). Biosimilars [mdash] why terminology matters.Nature biotechnology, 29(8), 690–693.

Westhovens, R., Yocum, D., Han, J., Berman, A., Strusberg, I., Geusens, P., & Rahman, M. U. (2006). The safety of infliximab, combined with background treatments, among patients with rheumatoid arthritis and various comorbidities: a large, randomized, placebo-controlled trial. Arthritis & Rheumatism, 54(4), 1075–1086.

Williams, R. O., Feldmann, M., & Maini, R. N. (1992). Anti-tumor necrosis factor ameliorates joint disease in murine collagen-induced arthritis.Proceedings of the National Academy of Sciences, 89(20), 9784–9788.

Winter, T. A., Wright, J., Ghosh, S., Jahnsen, J., Innes, A., & Round, P. (2004). Intravenous CDP870, a PEGylated Fab' fragment of a humanized antitumour necrosis factor antibody, in patients with moderate-to-severe Crohn's disease: an exploratory study. Alimentary pharmacology & therapeutics, 20(11-12), 1337–1346.

Wolfe, F., & Michaud, K. (2007). Biologic treatment of rheumatoid arthritis and the risk of malignancy: analyses from a large US observational study. Arthritis & Rheumatism, 56(9), 2886–2895

World Health Organization. (2004). The global burden of disease: 2004 update Retrieved from: http://www.who.int/healthinfo/global_burden_disease/2004_ report_update; accessed on 19th June 2014

Zhang, B., Combe, B., Rincheval, N., & Felson, D. T. (2012). Validation of ACR/EULAR definition of remission in rheumatoid arthritis from RA practice: the ESPOIR cohort. Arthritis Res Ther, 14, R156.

Zink A, Manger B, Kaufmann J, et al. Evaluation of the RABBIT Risk Score for serious Infections. Ann Rheum Dis Published Online First: [5th June 2013] doi:10.1136/annrheumdis-2013-203341

Zink, A., Askling, J., Dixon, W. G., Klareskog, L., Silman, A. J., & Symmons, D. P. M. (2009). European biologicals registers: methodology, selected results and perspectives. Annals of the rheumatic diseases, 68(8), 1240–1246.

Zuñiga, L., & Calvo, B. (2010). Biosimilars approval process. Regulatory Toxicology and Pharmacology, 56(3), 374–377.

Chapter 5

The Effect of Fluorocitrate at the Spinal Level in a Rat Monoarthritic Pain Model: Possible Modulatory Role of D-serine

Mariana Quiroz-Munoz[1], Alejandro Hernandez[2], Teresa Pelissier[3] and Claudio Laurido[2]

1 Introduction

Chronic pain is a clinical problem difficult to solve due to the incomplete knowledge we have about the adaptive changes that occurs in the neural substrates of the nociceptive system and glial cells in response to episodes of persistent pain. N-methyl Aspartate (NMDA) receptor antagonists inhibit the hyperexcitability of nociceptive neurons in the spinal cord induced by stimulation of C fibers (Davies & Lodge, 1987; Dickenson & Sullivan, 1987). This receptor is important in the establishment of chronic pain; furthermore, we know other factors that may modulate this pain, such as glial cells (Milligan & Watkins, 2009). Fluorocitrate (FC) is a specific inhibitor of glial metabolism. The application of 0.001 μM of FC administered intrastriatally in the rat causes a 95% reduction of glutamine formation from acetate, a substrate that permeates astrocyte cells selectively (Hassel et al., 1992). Glutamine is synthesized by astrocytes and constitutes an important precursor for the synthesis of glutamate and GABA, both in vitro and in vivo. FC also blocks the Krebs cycle enzyme aconitase in the astrocytes, dramatically decreasing the production of ATP (Serres et al., 2008) "shutting down" them metabolically and thus

[1] Laboratory of Renal Physiology, Faculty of Biological Sciences, Catholic University of Chile, Chile
[2] Department of Biology, Department of Biology, Faculty of Chemistry and Biology, University of Santiago of Chile, Chile
[3] ICBM, University of Chile, Chile

preventing the synthesis, among others, of proinflammatory cytokines (Guo *et al.*, 2007). Furthermore, FC (also minocycline, and SB203580) effectively inhibited IL-1b–induced reactive astrocytosis, microgliosis, and thermal hyperalgesia (Sung *et al.*, 2012). In this context, the exogenous application of D-serine should restitute their levels and concomitant to this, the nociceptive neuronal function.

2   Material and Methods

Experiments were carried out in 60 adults Sprague-Dawley (250–300 g) rats, normal and monoarthritic. The experiments presented in this work were performed according to the Ethics Committee of the University of Santiago of Chile and the Ethical Guidelines for Research on Experimental Pain in Conscious Animals (Zimmermann, 1983). In order to minimize the unnecessary suffering of animals, we utilized a maximum of six animals in each experiment. They were kept in a chamber with controlled temperature (25 °C ± 2) and light/dark cycles of 12/12 hours, starting at 8:00 AM, with food and water *ad libitum*.

2.1   Experimental Groups

Three groups of animals were prepared: rats injected with saline (saline means Artificial Cerebrospinal Fluid. It consists of two separate solutions. The first solution was composed of 7.597 g of NaCl, 0.231 g of KC1, 0.203 g of $MgCl_2$, 2.058 g of $NaHCO_3$, 0.69 g of NaH_2PO_4, and 500 ml of H_2O. The second solution was prepared with 5.376 g of glucose, 0.175 g of $CaCl_2$, and 500 ml of H_2O. Then the two solutions are mixed together) (Nakamura *et al.*, 1987) or FC, 0.002 µM at time zero and then tested as follows:

a) Normal rats injected with saline at time zero, 15, 30, 45, 60, 120, 240 and 360 minutes. (n = 6 rats)

   1. Monoarthritic rats injected with saline at time zero, 15, 30, 45, 60, 120, 240 and 360 minutes. (n = 6 rats)

   2. Normal rats injected with FC at time zero, 15, 30, 45, 60, 120, 240 and 360 minutes. (n = 6 rats)

   3. Monoarthritic rats injected with FC at time zero, 15, 30, 45, 60, 120, 240 and 360 minutes. (n = 6 rats)

b) Rats injected with saline or FC, 0.002 µM i.t. at time zero and then tested as follows:

   1. Normal rats injected with saline and tested at time zero, 15, 30, 45, 60, 90 and 120 minutes. (n = 6 rats)

   2. Normal rats injected with FC at time zero and submitted to spinal wind-up at times zero, 15, 30, 45 and 60 minutes. At time 60 minutes D-serine (300 µM) was injected and tested at times 60, 90 and 120 minutes. (n = 6 rats)

   3. Normal rats injected with FC at time zero and tested at time zero, 15, 30, 45,

60, 90 and 120 minutes. (n = 6 rats)

c) Rats injected with saline or FC, 0.002 μM i.t. at time zero and then tested as fol-
    lows:

1. Monoarthritic rats injected with saline and tested at time zero, 15, 30, 45, 60,
    90 and 120 minutes. (n = 6 rats)

2. Monoarthritic rats injected with FC at time zero and submitted to spinal
    wind-up at times zero, 15, 30, 45 and 60 minutes. At time 60 minutes D-
    serine (300 μM) was injected and tested at times 60, 90 and 120 minutes.
    (n = 6 rats)

3. Monoarthritic rats injected with FC at time zero and tested at time zero, 15,
    30, 45, 60, 90 and 120 minutes. (n = 6 rats)

Intrathecal administration of drugs was performed by percutaneous injections,
according to the method described by Mestre *et al.* (Mestre *et al*, 1994). Briefly, the i.t.
injection consist of administering either saline, FC or D-serine into the subarachnoid
space between lumbar vertebrae L5 and L6, using a Hamilton syringe with a needle 26G
× 1/2" in a maximum volume of 10 μL. To assure the needle has penetrated into the subarachnoid space, a slight movement in the tail of the rat occurs as a result of the needle
mechanical stimulation penetrating the meninges of the spinal cord.

Chemicals: D-serine was obtained from Sigma-Aldrich and dissolved in saline.
Fluorocitrate (Sigma-Aldrich) was prepared from barium fluorocitrate. Freund's complete adjuvant (Difco Lab.), experimental arthritis inductor. Briefly: 300 μg of *Mycobacterium butiricum* suspended in 0.6 ml of paraffin, 0.4 ml NaCl, 0.9% and 0.1 ml Tween 80,
injected in one intra articular bolus of 50 μL.

2.2   Experimental Model of Chronic Pain

Monoarthritis: This model of pathological pain was described by Butler *et al.*, (Bendele,
2001). Briefly, rats weighing 120–150 g approximately are inoculated with 50 μL of
complete Freund's adjuvant containing 300 μg of *Mycobacterium butiricum* in the right
ankle joint. This injection causes a localized arthritis syndrome, proving to be stable between four and six weeks post inoculation, establishing a persistent pain in the presence
of neurogenic hyperalgesia. This arthritic model has been used in preclinical testing of
numerous anti arthritic agents (Laurido *et al.*, 2003). It is maintained for a period exceed-
ing two months.

2.3   Electrophysiological Determinations

Spinal wind-up: The C fibers reflex was assessed in the normal and monoarthritic paw
using rats anesthetized with urethane (1g/Kg i.p.). Initially, C fibers were stimulated by
electrical shocks applied to the fourth and fifth toes of the hind paw, (territory innervat-
ed by the sural nerve), by means of two stainless steel electrodes. An intensity of 6–10
mA, duration of 2 ms and a frequency of 0.1 Hz is enough to evoke an electromyo-

graphic (EMG) activity. This EMG is recorded from the ipsilateral *biceps femoris* (Laurido *et al.*, 2003) by means of two stainless steel electrodes placed inside the muscle. This stimulation is maintained for around 20 minutes to allow stabilization of the response. Then, the threshold of stimulation is sought by diminishing the amplitude of stimulation until one half of the EMG elicits an electrical response and the other half don't. The values obtained for the C-fiber activation was shown in Table 1.

	Saline	FC, 0.002 μM
Normal rats	6.0 ± 0.8	9.1 ± 1.1‡
Monoarthritic rats	3.2 ± 0.3*	8.2 ± 0.9‡

Table 1: The table shows the stimulant current required for the threshold activation of the C-fiber evoked responses in normal and monoarthritic rats treated with FC or saline.

Values are means ± standard error of the mean of stimulating current required (in mA) in the normal and FC-treated rats for the C-fiber activation. Two-way analysis of variance (ANOVA) identified the FC treatment and the monoarthritic condition as significant factors influencing the stimulating current required for threshold activation of the C-reflex. No FC treatment × monoarthritic condition interaction was observed. Significant differences ($P < 0.01$) between FC-treated and saline-treated groups are denoted by ‡, while significant differences between monoarthritic and normal groups ($P < 0.01$) are indicated by an asterisk (according to the Bonferroni post hoc test). $n = 6$ animals in each group.

Then, stimulation at 0.1 Hz with intensity twice the threshold was maintained throughout the experiment as seen in Figure 1. In order to obtain the electromyographic response, the cumulative integral with a duration of 300 ms, (which corresponds to a time interval of 150–450 ms after the stimulus), was obtained for each stimulus. The maximum value of this integral corresponds to the electromyographic response (Figure 1, lower panel). It can be observed that the integral values are stable (between 0.025–0.034 V.s). These responses were fed into a computer equipped with a digital to analog converter (Powerlab/4S), and processed with the Chart 5.0 software. To evoke synaptic potentiation or wind-up, twelve stimuli at 1.0 Hz were applied.

Figure 2 shows a representative record of stimulation showing the resultant EMG (upper panel). The wind-up is observed as a synaptic potentiation manifested for the progressive increase in the number of muscle action potentials produced by the stimulation. This enhancement is verified up to the stimulus number 9, and later a decrease is observed. This decrease was associated with activation of descending inhibitory mechanisms from supraspinal structures. The lower part shows the cumulative integral with a duration of 300 ms, which corresponds to a time of 150–450 ms after the stimulus. This initial test was the control. After injecting FC or D-serine, the maximum values of each stimulus (only those that show an increasing trend, usually between the seventh to

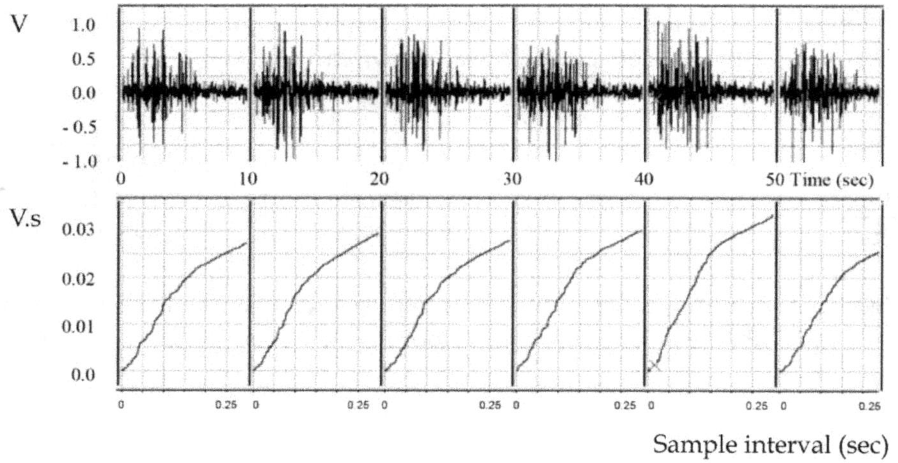

Figure 1: Representative electromyogram and cumulative integral of the C-reflex response.

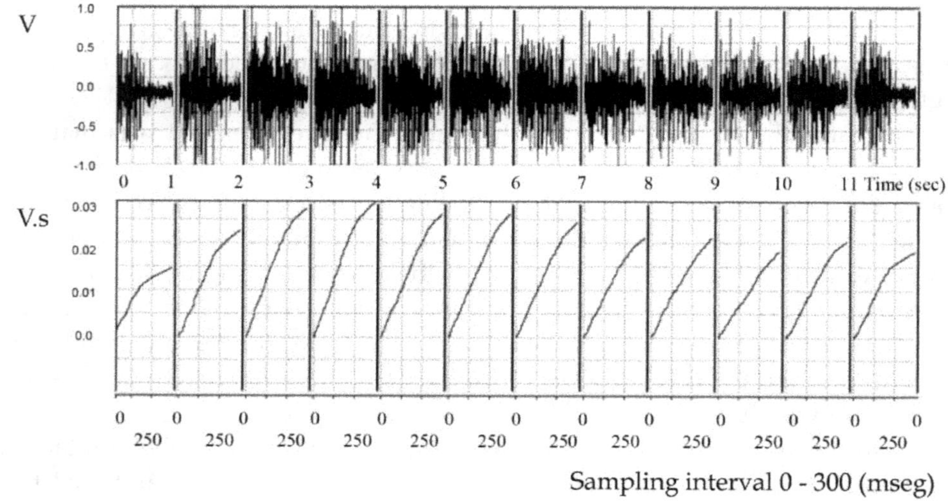

Figure 2: Representative electromyogram and cumulative integral of the spinal wind-up response.

eighth stimuli) were used and the slope was expressed as a percentage with respect to the normal animals (Laurido *et al.*, 2001). The results were expressed as mean ± SEM. $n = 6$ rats per experiment. * $P < 0.05$ according to one way ANOVA.

The upper part shows a representative electromyogram with stimulation at 0.1 Hz. In order to obtain only the C-fiber activity, a time window of 300 ms is set. This window starts at 150 ms after the stimulus. This allows us to collect all the C-fiber activity discarding other responses such as Aδ fiber activity. The lower part shows the cumulative integral of the C-reflex responses. The maximum values of the sampling interval correspond to the C-reflex response for each time. This figure is valid for normal and monoarthritic rats. The only difference is the activation threshold for evoking the C-fiber evoked responses as shown in Table 1.

Electromyogram (upper part) and their associate integral (lower part). The sampling frequency is increased to 1 Hz in order to induce the C-fiber potentiation. Each sampling interval corresponds to a time window of 300 ms of duration, initiated 150 ms after the stimulus. This sample collects all the C-fiber activity discarding other responses such as Aδ fiber activity. The lower part shows the cumulative integral of the C-reflex responses. The C-fiber potentiation can be seen during the first four time intervals, where the integral increases the Vs value (from around 0.03 to 0.06 V.s). The slopes of the maximum of these four values correspond to the Wind-up response. This figure is valid for normal and monoarthritic rats. The only difference is the activation threshold for evoking the wind-up as shown in Table 1.

3   Results

Figure 3 shows the effect of FC applied to normal and monoarthritic rats at time zero. It can be observed that the antinociceptive effect of FC is maintained on time, reaching a plateau for both rats at around 120 minutes and sustained over the time until at least 360 minutes of testing. No longer times were attempted since that test is invasive in the sense that electrodes are placed into the muscle tissue and inside the toes, and might produce local inflammatory problems in the interface tissue electrode, altering the results.

Effect of saline on normal (S NR) and monoarthritic (S MR) rats: FC 0.002 μM was i.t. applied at time zero to both normal (FC NR) and monoarthritic (FC MR) rats. It can be seen that the antinociceptive effect spans at even 360 minutes. No longer times were tested (see text). $n = 6$, number of rats for each series of experiments.

Effect of saline, D-serine and FC on the spinal cord wind-up on normal rats: Figure 4 shows the effect of FC and D-serine in the wind-up cord of normal rats. At time zero was injected saline i.t. to the rats. The wind-up in rats with saline (black column, Saline Normal Rat (NR)) did not produce any significant change or was slightly algesic from zero to 120 minutes. A second series of experiments were done. FC was applied at time zero and the development of antinociception was followed at times 15, 30, 45, 60, 90 and 120 minutes (Green, FC Normal Rat (NR)). It can be observed that there is an increment in the antinociception over time, reaching a maximum of around 60 minutes,

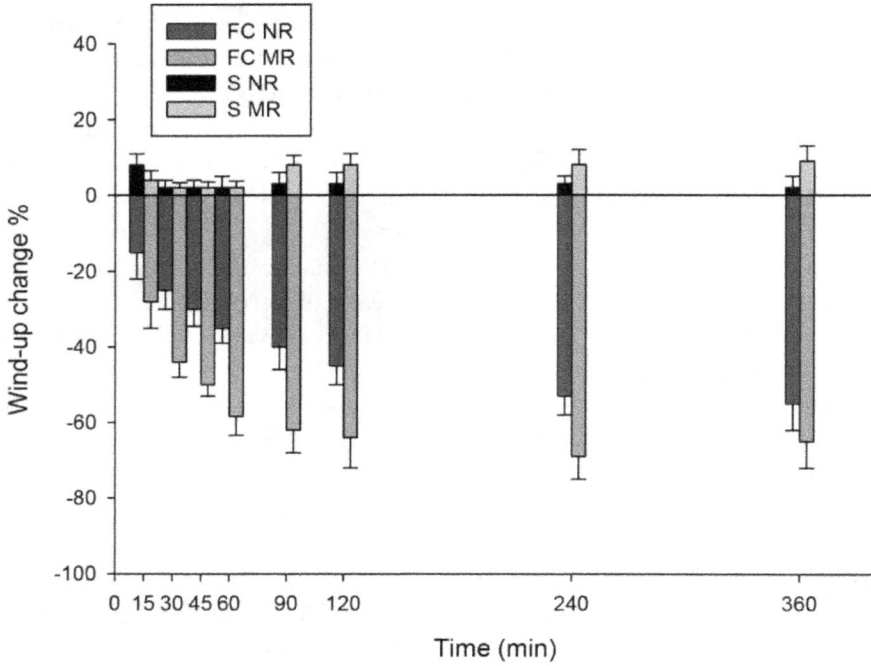

Figure 3: Time course of the effect of FC alone on normal and monoarthritic rats.

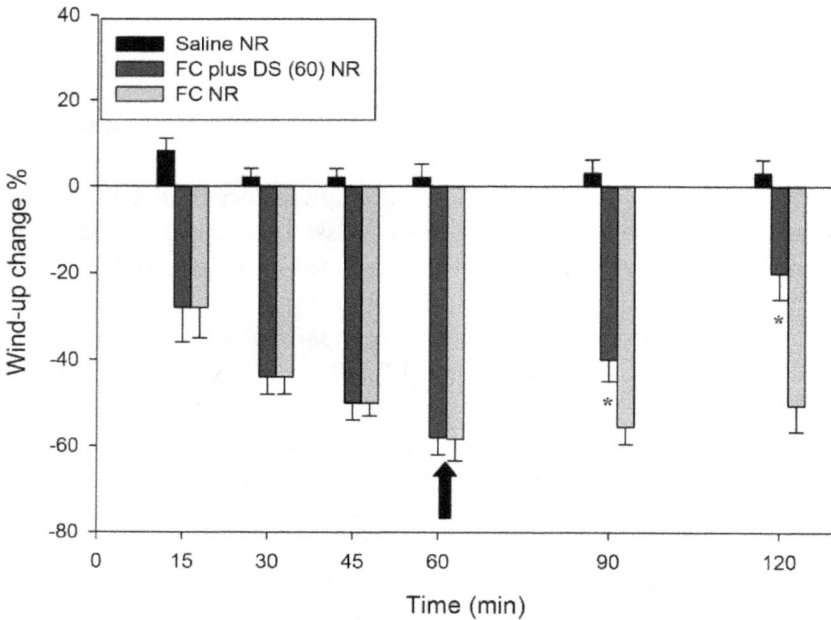

Figure 4: Effect of saline, FC and D-serine in the wind-up cord of normal rats.

and then maintained up to 120 minutes. A third series of experiments were done. (Red, FC plus DS (60) NR). FC was applied at time zero observing a development of antinociception very similar to the one of FC alone. At time 60 minutes, D-serine (300 µM i.t., black arrow) was injected and the wind-up measured at times 90 and 120 minutes. It can be observed that there is a decrease in the antinociception (around 65%, at 90 minutes and 34% at 120 minutes) statistically significant ($P < 0.05$) for both times when compared with the time 60 minutes.

Effect of saline (black column, Saline Normal Rat (NR)): FC was applied at time zero and the development of antinociception was followed at times 15, 30, 45, 60, 90 and 120 minutes; In the green bar, FC Normal Rat (NR), FC was applied at time zero observing a development of antinociception very similar to the one of FC alone. At time 60 minutes, D-serine (300 µM i.t., black arrow) was injected and the wind-up measured at times 90 and 120 minutes. (Red column, FC plus DS (60) Normal Rat (NR)). $n = 6$, number of rats for each series of experiments. * = $p < 0.05$ according to one way ANOVA.

Effect of saline, D-serine and FC on the spinal cord wind-up on monoarthritic rats: Essentially, the same results as the normal ones appear in the monoarthritic rats. Figure 5 shows the effect of the application of saline at time zero (Black column, Saline Monoarthritic Rat). It can be observed that the effect of saline is more pronounced that the same treatment for normal rats. A second series of experiments were done. FC was applied at time zero and the development of antinociception was followed at times 15, 30, 45, 60, 90 and 120 minutes (Green, FC Monoarthritic Rat (MR)). It can be observed that there is an increment in the antinociception over time, which is maintained up to 120 minutes. A third series of experiments were done. (Red, FC plus DS (60) MR). FC was applied at time zero observing a development of antinociception very similar to the one of FC alone. At time 60 minutes, D-serine (300 µM i.t. black arrow) was injected and the wind-up measured at times 90 and 120 minutes. It can be observed that there is a decrease in the antinociception, around 50 %, at 90 minutes and 80% at 120 minutes) statistically significant ($P < 0.05$) for both times, when compared with the time 60 minutes.

Effect of saline (black column, Saline Monoarthritic Rat (MR)): FC was applied at time zero and the development of antinociception was followed at times 15, 30, 45, 60, 90 and 120 minutes (Green, FC Monoarthritic Rat (MR)); FC was applied at time zero observing a development of antinociception very similar to the one of FC alone. At time 60 minutes, D-serine (300 µM i.t., black arrow) was injected and the wind-up measured at times 90 and 120 minutes. (Red, FC plus DS (60) Monoarthritic Rat (MR)). $n = 6$, number of rats for each series of experiments. * = $p < 0.05$ according to one way ANOVA.

4   Discussion

The results obtained in this work showed that the analgesic effect of FC i.t. injected into normal rats or those presenting an experimental model of arthritis, can be possibly modulated by the i.t administration of D-serine. These experiments were done using the spinal wind-up as a test for nociception. Electrical stimulation of the leg is a very suita-

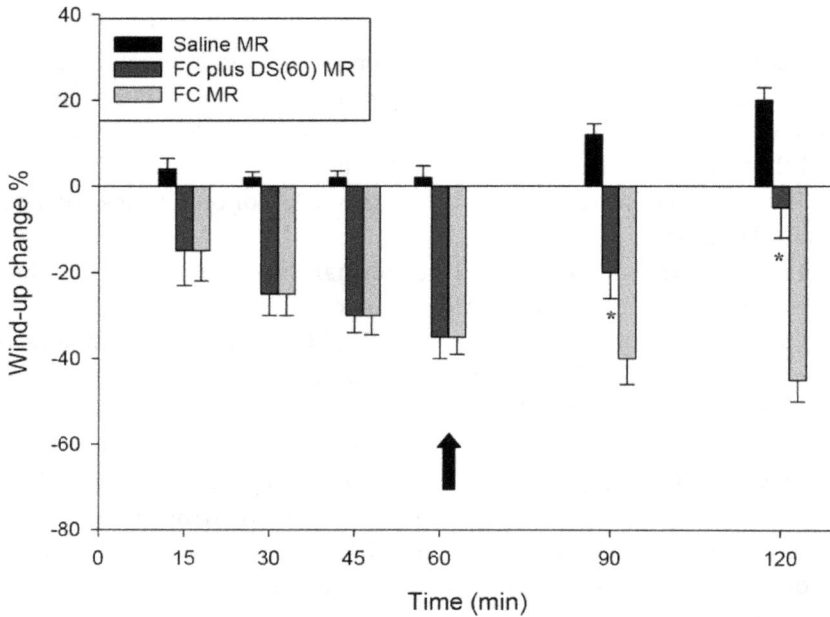

Figure 5: Effect of saline, FC and D-serine in the wind-up cord of monoarthritic rats

ble assay to quantify the effect of drugs, since it constitutes a demanding test requiring the action of very efficient antinociceptive drugs to achieve a notable or statistically significant effect. This test triggers nociceptive fibers that can be isolated because of his speed, allowing us to have mainly a C-fiber reflex response. The C-fiber response to electrical stimulation provides objective parameters of nociception. This is advantageous compared to behavioral approaches in which there is a subjective assessment of pain-like responses.

There is abundant evidence that glial cells are crucial to produce hyperalgesia/allodynia, which eventually generates the central sensitization phenomena, establishing the pain as a chronic condition and usually resistant to a number of anti-inflammatory drugs and analgesics used as first-line treatment for acute pain (Scholz & Clifford, 2007). Previous reports indicate that the nociceptive response in several animal models of chronic pain is attenuated due to inactivation of the glia or by preventing the action of pro-inflammatory cytokines (Watkins & Maier, 2003). For example, the chronic administration of intrathecal propentofylline reduces mechanical allodynia in a neuropathic pain model using von Frey filaments to assess the nociceptive response to tactile stimuli (Obata *et al.*, 2010). FC has been used to reduce formalin-induced hyperalgesia and mechanical allodynia induced neuropathy produced by sciatic nerve inflammation (Watkins & Maier, 2002). Electro acupuncture has been used also as an antagonizing agent in thermal hyperalgesia and mechanical allodynia induced in the paw by adjuvant induced arthritis. The use of FC has helped to produce a synergistic effect enhancing the analgesia induced by electro acupuncture (Sun *et al.*, 2006). The antinociceptive action of FC can be attributed to the metabolic and functional inhibition of the astrocytes located in the spinal cord. Once the astrocytes are activated under physiopathological conditions such as inflammation, neuropathies or oncological pain, these cells are capable of release into the extracellular media, pro inflammatory cytokines and other neuromodulators such as ATP. These substances could affect the second order neurons favoring the glutamate pathway mediated by the NMDA receptors. One of these substances is D-serine. D-serine is an endogenous ligand for the glycine site of the NMDA receptor (Mothet *et al.*, 2000) and represents an important new source of modulation of glial brain cells. FC also inhibits the up-regulation of NOS expression, activity and production in the spinal cord, induced by the formalin test in rats (Sun *et al.*, 2009). D-serine in the brain of the rat cerebral cortex is enriched in the rostral hippocampus, anterior olfactory nucleus, striatum and amygdala. In addition, D-serine has been found in the vertebrate retina (Stevens *et al.*, 2003). On the role of D-serine in pain, D-serine has a pronociceptive effect when applied intrathecally. D-serine produces a facilitation of the rat tail flick, and is blocked by co administration of 7-chlorokynurenic acid (Kolhekar *et al.*, 1994). D-serine levels can be modified by inhibiting the racemization of L-serine by the serine racemase inhibitors, L-Serine-O-Sulfate (LSOS), and L-Erythro-3-Hydroxyaspartate. Both compounds injected intrathecally decreased the wind-up in normal and monoarthritic rats. Interestingly, the antinociceptive effect was abolished when 300 µg/10 µL was injected intrathecally (Laurido *et al.*, 2012). On the other hand, in dynamic mechanical allodynia (DMA) (from rat chronic infraorbital nerve constriction), the astrocytes play a role in the synthesis of D-serine, since the administration of LSOS decreased pain behavior in allodynic rats. Administration of FC alleviated DMA, indicating a role of astrocytes since this compound block astrocyte metabolism, (Dieb & Hafidi, 2013) situation similar to the results found in this work for normal and monoarthritic rats.

5   Conclusions

These results may have applications in the knowledge of the mechanisms involved in the maintenance of chronic pain, in conditions were chronic pain is poorly controlled by drugs currently in use. In conclusion, the prevention of spinal glial activation by FC may not only alleviate the early symptoms of a disease, but also prevent, for example, the development of opioid dependence, increasing the possibility of maintaining prolonged pain relief.

Acknowledgements

This study was supported by grants from DICYT 011043LF, 021343LF and 021643LF, University of Santiago of Chile.

References

Bendele, A. M. (2001) Animal models of osteoarthritis. Journal of Musculoskeletical & Neuronal Interactions, 1(4), 363–76.

Butler, S.H., Godefroy, F., Besson, J.M. & Weil-Fugazza, J. (1992) A limited arthritic model studies in a model of monoarthritis in the rat. Pain, 48, 73–81.

Davies, S. N. & Lodge, D. (1987) Evidence for involvement of N-Methylaspartate receptor in "wind-up" of class 2 neurones in the dorsal horn of the rat". Brain Research, 424, 402–6.

Dickenson, A. H. & Sullivan, A.F. (1987) Evidence for a role of the NMDA receptor in the frequency dependent potentiation of deep rat dorsal horn nociceptive neurones following C fibre stimulation. Neuropharmacology, 26, 1235–8, 1987.

Dieb, W. & Hafidi, A. (2013) Astrocytes are involved in trigeminal dynamic mechanical Allodynia potential role of D-serine. Journal of Dental Research 92(9), 808–813.

Guo, W., Wang, H., Watanabe, M., Shimizu, K., Zou, S., LaGraize, S. C., Wei, F., Dubner, R. & Ren, K. (2007) Glial–Cytokine–Neuronal Interactions Underlying the Mechanisms of Persistent Pain. Journal of Neuroscience, 27(2), 6006–6018.

Hassel, B., Paulsen, R.E., Johnsen, A. & Fonnum, F. (1992) Selective inhibition of glial cell metabolism in vivo by fluorocitrate. Brain Research, 576,120–124.

Kolhekar, R., Meller S.T. & Gebhart, G.F. (1994) N-methyl-D-aspartate receptor-mediated changes in thermal nociception: allosteric modulation at glycine and polyamine recognition sites. Neuroscience, 63(4), 925–36.

Laurido, C., Hernández, A., Constandil, L., & Pelissier, T. (2003) Nitric oxide synthase and soluble guanylate cyclase are involved in spinal cord wind-up activity of monoarthritic, but not of normal rats. Neuroscience Letters, 352, 64–66.

Laurido, C., Hernandez, A., Pelissier, T. & Constandil, L. (2012) Antinociceptive Effect of Rat D-Serine Racemase Inhibitors, L-Serine-O-Sulfate, and L-Erythro-3-Hydroxyaspartate in an Arthritic Pain Model. The Scientific World Journal vol. 2012, Article ID 279147, 5 pages.

Laurido, C., Pelissier, T., Pérez, H., Flores, F. & Hernández, A. (2001) Effect of ketamine on spinal cord nociceptive transmission in normal and monoarthritic rats. NeuroReport, 12, 551–1554.

Mestre, C., Pelissier, T., Fialip, J., Wilcox, G. & Eschalier, A. (1994) A method to perform direct transcutaneous intrathecal injection in rats. Journal of Pharmacological and Toxicological Methods, 32, 197–200.

Milligan, E. D. & Watkins, L.R. Pathological and protective roles of glia in chronic pain. (2009) Nature Neuroscience, 10, p 23–36.

Mothet, J.P., Parent, A.T., Wolosker, H., Brady Jr, R.O., Linden, D.J., Ferris, C.D. & Snyder, S.H. (2000) D-serine is an endogenous ligand for the glycine site of the N-methyl-D-aspartate receptor. Proceedings of the Natural Academy of Sciences. USA. 97(9), 4926–31,

2000.

Nakamura, K., Osborn Jr, J.W. & Cowley Jr., A.W. (1987) *Pressor response to small elevations of cerebroventricular pressure in conscious rats.* Hypertension, 10, 635–641.

Obata, H., Sakurazawa, S., Kimura, M., Saito, S. (2010) *Activation of astrocytes in the spinal cord contributes to the development of bilateral allodynia after peripheral nerve injury in rats.* Brain Research, 1363, 72–80.

Scholz, J. & Clifford, C.J. (2007) *The neuropathic pain triad: neurons, immune cells and glia.* Nature Neurosciences, 10(11), 1361–1368.

Serres, S., Raffard, G., Franconi, M. & Merle, M. (2008) *Close coupling between astrocytic and neuronal metabolisms to fulfill anaplerotic and energy needs in the rat brain.* Journal of Cerebral Blood Flow Metabolism, 28, 712–724.

Stevens, E.R., Esguerra, M., Kim, M.P.M., Newman, E.A., Snyder, S.H., Zahs, K.R. & Miller, R.F. (2003) *D-serine and serine racemase are present in the vertebrate retina and contribute to the physiological activation of NMDA receptors.* Proceedings of the Natural Academy of Sciences, USA, 100, 6789–6794.

Sun, S., Chen, W.L., Wang, P.F., Zhao, Z.Q. & Zhang, Y.Q. (2006) *Disruption of glial function enhances electroacupuncture analgesia in arthritic rats.* Experimental Neurology, 198, 294–302.

Sun, X. C., Chen, W. N., Li, S.Q., Cai, J.S., Li, W. B., Xian, X.H., Hu, Y.Y., Zhang, M., & Li, Q.J. (2009) *Fluorocitrate, an inhibitor of glial metabolism, inhibits the Up-regulation of NOS expression, activity and NO production in the spinal cord induced by formalin test in rats.* Neurochemical Research. 34(2), 351–359.

Sung, C-S., Cherng, C-H., Wen, Z-H., Chang, W-K, Huang, S-Y, Lin, S-L, Chan, K-H & Wong, C-S. (2012) *Minocycline and Fluorocitrate Suppress Spinal Nociceptive Signaling in Intrathecal IL-1b–Induced Thermal Hyperalgesic Rats.* Glia, 60, 2004–2017.

Watkins, L. & Maier, S. (2002) *Beyond neurons: evidence that immune and glial cells contribute to pathological pain states.* Physiological Reviews, 82, 981–1011.

Watkins, L. & Maier, S. (2003) *Glia: a novel drug discovery target for clinical pain.* Nature Review Drug Discovery, 2(12), 973–985.

Zimmermann, M. (1983) *Ethical guidelines for investigations of experimental pain in conscious animals.* Pain, 16, 109–110.

Chapter 6

Lean Type 2 Diabetes Mellitus

Keisam Reetu Devi[1], Manash Pratim Baruah[2], Salam Ranabir[3]

1 Introduction

Type 2 diabetes is increasing in epidemic proportions across the globe. Obesity is gener-ally considered to be the major contributor to the epidemic of diabetes mellitus. In NHANES 1999–2002 study from USA around 55% of diabetics were obese (Eberhardt & Ogden, 2004) The focus in the Western world remains on the more prevalent over-weight or obese patient, but a significant proportion of diabetes cannot be attributable to obesity using current criteria. A large proportion of patients with type 2 diabetes are 'lean or underweight.' In the Diabetes and Informatics (DAI) study in Italy involving over 13,000 patients with type 2 diabetes, approximately 25% had a body mass index (BMI) $\leq$ 25 kg/m^2 and rates of obesity were 23% in men and 37% in women (Mannucci *et al*. 2004). Likewise, in a study involving over 2700 people with type 2 diabetes attending a secondary care diabetes clinic in the UK, 14% had a BMI $\leq$ 25 kg/m^2 and 52% were Obese (Daousi & Casson, 2006).

There is some controversy, however, as to what exactly defines a lean patient with type 2 diabetes. There is uncertainty regarding the choice of the most appropriate parameters and their thresholds for defining overweight and obesity, the influence of different patient characteristics, such as ethnicity and age (National Heart, Lung, and Blood Institute Expert Panel on the Identification, Evaluation, and Treatment of Over-weight and Obesity in Adults, 1998). In South Asians, people who are not overweight by traditional weight criteria (i.e. BMI) may have an increased percentage of body fat, particularly the more metabolically active intra-abdominal fat (Deurenberg-Yap *et al.*,

---

[1] Department of Physiology, Jawaharlal Nehru Institute of Medical Sciences, Imphal, India

[2] Division of Endocrinology, Excel Centre, Guwahati, India

[3] Department of Medicine, Regional Institute of medical Sciences, Imphal, India

2000; Vikram *et al.*, 2003). For the same level of waist circumference compared with Caucasians, Japanese subjects have a larger mass of adipose tissue (Kadowaki *et al.*, 2006).

Thus, when considering whether a person with type 2 diabetes is 'lean', several factors need to be considered, including BMI, waist circumference and ethnicity; and appropriate threshold values should be used. International Diabetes Federation (IDF) have set a separate cut-off for anthropometric parameters for South Asians distinct from the Caucasians (Alberti *et al.*, 2006).

2   Prevalence

In 1965 Tripathy and Kar from India highlighted the fact that 27% of elderly diabetics were lean (Tripathy & Kar, 1965). Several other studies from India also have reported a prevalence rate of lean diabetes ranging from 3.5%–18.1% (Chaudhary *et al.*, 2013; Das *et al.*, 1995; Mohan *et al.*, 1997; Mukhyaprana *et al.*, 2004).

In NHANES 1999–2002 study from USA around 15% of diabetics were lean, although in this study the diabetics were not categorized into type 1 or type 2 (Eberhardt & Ogden, 2004).

At the Cook County Diabetes Center (CCDC), serving minority population in Chicago, 13% of 18,000 patients with diabetes mellitus were lean (BMI < 25 but > 17 kg/m²) (Coleman *et al.*, 2014)

There are also several studies reporting lean type 2 diabetes from many Asian countries. In a study from China, 5.8% of newly referred type 2 diabetics were lean using a BMI cut-off of 18.5 kg/m² (Chan *et al.*, 2004). In another study from China of 1000 type 2 diabetic patients, 58% had a BMI less than 25 kg/m² (Taniguchi *et al.*, 2000). A Japanese study of 111 untreated type 2 diabetes reported 8% of the patients were lean using a BMI cut-off of 21.5 kg/m² (Lu *et al.*, 2006). The preferred cut-off for Asians/Indians to define as lean or underweight is a BMI of 18.5 kg/m2 (International Diabetes Institute, 2000).

3   Risk factors

In a study from US which compared lean diabetes patients to their obese counterparts, 56% of lean patients reported having a first degree relative with diabetes compared to 62% in the obese diabetes group ($p < 0.001$). In the lean group, 30.5% were current smokers and 5.7% had a history of alcoholism compared to 22% and 2.4%, respectively, in the obese population ($p < 0.001$). There was a higher prevalence of pancreatitis: 3.6% in the lean diabetics compared to 0.9% in obese patients ($p < 0.001$) (Coleman *et al.*, 2014).

A region on chromosome 21q has been identified to contribute to type 2 diabetes mellitus in lean individuals (Iwasaki *et al.*, 2003). Further examination of this region led to the identification of KCNJ15 (potassium inwardly-rectifying channel, subfamily J, member 15) as a susceptibility gene (Okamoto *et al.*, 2010). KCNJ15 is linked to dysfunctional glucose-stimulated insulin secretion (GSIS) in lean Japanese patients with type 2 diabetes (Okamoto *et al.*, 2012). Other studies have also shown that lean type 2 diabetics have a stronger genetic predisposition. A variant (rs8090011) in the LAMA1 gene was more strongly associated with type 2 diabetes in lean cases than in obese cases (Perry *et al.*, 2012). TCF7L2 also has a stronger effect in non-obese cases compared to obese cases (Tsai *et al.*, 2010).

4   Pathophysiology

Normal weight people with type 2 diabetes often have better insulin sensitivity, but greater insulin secretory deficits, compared with overweight/obese patients. Nevertheless, some degree of insulin resistance is a frequent characteristic feature of normal weight people with type 2 diabetes (DeFronzo *et al.*, 2004). There are some reports of reduced glucose transporters in diabetics. Garvey *et al.* (1988) reported that the numbers as well as the intrinsic activity of glucose carriers are reduced in adipose tissue of obese Type 2 diabetic patients. Similarly there is a reduction in the number of GLUT 4 in the plasma membrane fraction of skeletal muscle of lean diabetic patients in the basal state (Vogt *et al.*, 1992). In contrast, Handberg *et al.* (1990) and Pedersen *et al.* (1990) did not find a significant alteration in the GLUT 4 number in human skeletal muscle of diabetic patients or control subjects in the basal state.

   Glucose storage is severely impaired in lean type 2 diabetes and a decrease in non-esterified fatty acid levels enhances muscle glucose oxidation and non-oxidative glycolysis but not glycogen synthesis. Changes in glycogen synthase action, which results in dysregulation of glucose storage in skeletal muscle after meal ingestion is probably the main alteration of glucose metabolism in lean type 2diabetic subjects (1996).

   Lean type 2 diabetics have been demonstrated to have a 41% deficit ($P < 0.05$) in relative β-cell volume compared with non-diabetic lean individuals. Obese type 2 diabetics have a 63% ($P < 0.01$) deficit in relative β-cell volume compared to non-diabetic obese subjects. Frequency of β-cell apoptosis is increased 10-fold in lean and 3-fold in obese type 2 diabetes compared with non-diabetic lean and obese individual respectively, ($P < 0.05$) (Butler *et al.*, 2003). Several studies have evaluated patients of lean type 2 diabetes using either clamps or homeostatic model assessment (HOMA). There are also studies where C-peptide is measured in basal state and/or after stimulation.

4.1   C-peptide Studies

Mohan *et al.* (1997) found no significant difference in the fasting or stimulated C-peptide levels between lean and obese diabetics. Diabetes in lean Japanese patients is associated with a low level of fasting insulin in addition to reduced peripheral glucose uptake and elevated endogenous glucose production (Takahara *et al.*, 2011). These data suggest that this disorder in normal-weight individual results from impaired insulin secretion and action.

Interestingly in the study by Das *et al.* (1995), mean basal insulin is lower in lean type 2 diabetics but there is no significant difference in basal C-peptide value compared to obese type 2 diabetics. Lean type 2 diabetics have a significantly lower rise in serum insulin level after oral glucose load as well as after 1mg IV glucagon compared to obese patients. But C-peptide did not differ significantly between the two types, suggesting similar reserve in beta cell function. The disparity between serum insulin and c-peptide level in lean type 2 diabetics may be due to greater extraction of insulin by liver. However, in another study by Das *et al.* (2007), mean values of fasting insulin and fasting C-peptide in lean and normal body weight individuals respectively did not differ significantly. Even though total proinsulin immunoreactivity (PIM) is significantly elevated in lean type 2 diabetic patients compared with lean control subjects, fasting insulin, c-peptide, ratio of intact proinsulin to PIM are comparable between the obese and lean type 2 diabetes. But after glucagon stimulation, PIM levels are significantly elevated in the diabetic subjects; more pronouncedly in the obese diabetic patients. The ratio of PIM to insulin or C-peptide during the test is significantly elevated in both lean and obese diabetic patients; more pronouncedly in the lean group (Roder *et al.*, 1999). In the study by Chan *et al.* (2004), serum C-peptide was lowest in the underweight and highest in overweight patients.

4.2   Clamp studies

In hyperinsulinemic euglycemic and hyperglycemic clamp study by Suraamornkul *et al.* (2010), lean patients had higher sensitivity to exogenous insulin. Insulin sensitivity was similar in lean type 2 diabetics compared to lean non-diabetic control subjects. First and second phase of insulin and C-peptide was significantly decreased in lean type 2 diabetics. Using the euglycemic insulin clamp with a D-[3-3H]glucose infusion 87.5% with a BMI less than 24.0 kg/m^2 were insulin sensitive, and 88.9% with a BMI greater than 28.5 kg/m^2 were insulin resistant (Banerji & Lebovitz, 1992).

Using hyperinsulinaemic euglycaemic clamp, diabetic patients with abdominal obesity has been shown to display peripheral insulin resistance in combination with defective insulin secretion, whereas non-obese diabetic patients showed only a secretory defect (Arner *et al.*, 1991). Visceral abdominal fat area measured by DXA correlates inversely with insulin sensitivity determined by glucose infusion rate during euglycemic hyperinsulinemic clamp in lean subjects independent of percent total body fat similar to obese type 2 diabetic subjects (Rattarasarn *et al.*, 2003).

In lean type 2 diabetics there is no impairment in hepatic but a slight reduction in extrahepatic insulin sensitivity but insulin release is markedly impaired (Pigon *et al.*, 1996). Leg glucose uptake and oxidation is similar in lean type 2 diabetics with age, sex and relative weight controls. The combine net balance of lactate and Ala is lower in lean type 2 diabetics. Basal muscle glycogen synthase is lower in lean subjects but activated to a similar extent during hyperinsulinemic clamp study (Kelly *et al.*, 1993).

4.3   Homeostasis Model Assessment Insulin Resistance (HOMA-IR)

HOMA-IR has consistently shown correlation to BMI. Eighty-eight percent of T2DM patients with a BMI ≤ 27.0 kg/m^2 were insulin-resistant, whereas 92% T2DM patients with a BMI < 21.5 kg/m^2 are insulin-sensitive. Type 2 diabetic patients with midrange BMI (21.5 to 27.0 kg/m^2), are equally likely to be insulin-resistant or insulin-sensitive (Taniguchi *et al.*, 2000). Lean type 2 DM demonstrated better beta cell function with homeostasis model assessment beta cells (HOMA-B) compared to normal body weight type 2 DM. Insulin resistance as assessed by HOMA- IR did not differ significantly between lean and normal body weight type 2 DM, suggesting that lean type 2 DM are actually a variant of the classic phenotype (Das *et al*, 2007). Moreover, HOMA-IR results were similar amongst underweight (< 18.5 kg/m^2), normal weight (18.5–23 kg/m^2) and overweight ($\geq$ 23 kg/m^2) (Chan *et al.*, 2004).

Another interesting facet of insulin-sensitive lean T2DM is normal non-insulin mediated glucose uptakes (NIMGU) but diminished glucose effectiveness at zero insulin (GEZI) (García-Estévez *et al.*, 2002). This may have important bearing on the clinical presentation of such a phenotype.

5   Autoantibodies Markers

Coleman *et al.* (2014) evaluated islet cell antibodies in 53 out of 1784 lean diabetic patients, of which 89% tested negative. In an Italian population-based cohort of 130 lean (BMI < 25 kg/m^2) patients with newly diagnosed diabetes approximately 50% tested positive for GAD and/or islet cell antibodies, suggesting that this phenotype may be highly prevalent among lean patients (Bruno *et al.*, 1999). In contrast to low reporting of anti-GADAb amongst lean T2DM by Mohan *et al.* (1997) of 9.6%, Unnikrishnan *et al.* (2004) reported a much higher prevalence (25.3%) for the same. In the study by Mohan *et al.* (1997) number of lean diabetics testing positive for anti-GADAb was not much higher than ideal body weight subjects (5.1%), or obese subjects (4.2%). Lean T2DM with anti-glutamic acid decarboxylase antibody (GADAb) positivity are younger and have lower beta cell function (HOMA-B) as compared to the GADAb-negative group, thus suggesting that the former group could have a slowly progressive form of type 1 diabetes or Latent autoimmune diabetes of adults (LADA) (Unnikrishnan *et al.*, 2004).

But as reported in several studies, vast majority of lean type 2 diabetes are antibody negative, (Bruno *et al.*, 1999; Mohan *et al.*, 1997; Unnikrishnan *et al.*, 2004) and their c-peptide level is not significantly different from obese type 2 diabetics (Das *et al.*, 1995; 2007; Mohan *et al.*, 1997) suggesting that they are a distinct clinical entity from LADA. Another differential diagnosis to be considered is maturity onset diabetes of the young (MODY) which typically have one or more of the following: a strong family history of diabetes, onset of diabetes in the second to fifth decade, insulin independence, absence of features of insulin resistance and absence of β-cell autoimmunity (Thanabalasingham & Owen, 2011).

6   Clinical features and Complications

6.1   Gender

There is a definite male preponderance in lean type 2 diabetes mellitus. (Arnab *et al.*, 2006; Coleman *et al.*, 2014; Das *et al.*, 1995; Mohan *et al.*, 1997; Mukhyaprana *et al.*, 2004; Punyakrit *et al.*, 2011) In contrast, 70% of obese diabetics were females, whereas 65% of lean diabetics were males in the study by Mukhyaparna *et al.* (2004) Coleman *et al.* (2014) working on US population 62% of lean T2DM were males. Among obese patients only 48% were male.

6.2   Age

As demonstrated by several Indian studies, mean age of lean T2DM ranges from 45–58 years (Das *et al.*, 1995; Mohan *et al.*, 1997; Mukhyaprana *et al.*, 2004; Punyakrit *et al.*, 2011). In the study from USA, the mean age of onset of lean type2 diabetes was 44 years which is similar to obese diabetics (Coleman *et al.*, 2014). Similarly, Mohan *et al.* (1997), did not observe any significant differences in the age at diagnosis among lean, ideal weight and obese type 2 diabetics. However in the study by Mukhyaparna *et al.* (2004), the mean age of onset of diabetes in lean diabetics was significantly higher compared to the mean for obese diabetics. But in the Thai study by Rattarasarn *et al.* (2003), the mean age of lean type 2 diabetics was lower than of obese type 2 diabetics, which of course, was not significantly different.

6.3   Glycemic Status

Mean fasting, post-prandial or 2 hr postchallenge blood glucose higher among lean patients (Das *et al.*, 1995; Mohan *et al.*, 1997; Mukhyaprana *et al.*, 2004). HbA1c level was also significantly higher in the lean group compared to obese (Chan *et al.*, 2004; Coleman *et al.*, 2014; Das *et al.*, 1995; Mohan *et al.*, 1997).

6.4   Blood Pressure

Hypertension was seen in 12% of lean type 2 diabetics (Punyakrit *et al.*, 2011). In another Indian study, incidence of hypertension in lean diabetics was 16.2%, whereas it was 39.09% in normal weight 41.6% in over weight and 61.5% in obese diabetics (Mukhyaprana *et al.*, 2004). Both systolic and diastolic blood pressure were significantly lower in the lean T2DM compared to ideal body weight and obese groups (Chan *et al.*, 2004; Mohan *et al.*, 1997). Coleman *et al.* (2014) also reported that lean diabetes patients had lower blood pressure compared to obese.

6.5   Lipid Profile

There is no gross abnormality in lipid profile among lean diabetics (Punyakrit *et al.*,

2011). Lipid profile was more favorable in lean diabetics compared to obese in some studies (Arnab *et al.*, 2006; Das *et al.*, 1995). Serum cholesterol and triglycerides levels were the lowest in the lean group and were progressively higher in the ideal body weight and obese groups ($P < 0.001$) (Mohan *et al.*, 1997). Serum triglyceride showed increasing, while HDL-C showed decreasing trends across different BMI groups (Chan *et al.*, 2004). Serum TG/HDL ratio was significantly lower in the lean as opposed to the obese T2DM subjects (Coleman *et al.*, 2014). Glycaemic control did not influence lipid metabolism in lean NIDDM patients, BMI < 25 kg/m^2 in men and < 27 kg/m^2 in women (Ikeda *et al.*, 1991).

6.6   Microvascular Complications

In the study by Punyakrit *et al.* (2011), from India, prevalence of peripheral neuropathy (70%) and retinopathy (25%) is higher among the lean diabetic patients as compared to macrovascular complications. Thirteen patients (13%) were suffering from nephropathy. Such a trend of higher prevalence of retinopathy among lean patients compared to ideal body weight and obese groups have been observed by others also. There was no significant difference in the occurrence of nephropathy between the groups. Among males with T2DM, peripheral neuropathy was more common in lean compared to obese, but no such difference was noted among females (Mohan *et al.*, 1997).

However, Mukhyaparna *et al.* (2004) did not find any difference in the prevalence of microvascular complications among lean, overweight and obese T2DM, something similar to a study from USA by Coleman *et al.* (2014)

6.7   Macrovascular Complication

The prevalence of macrovascular complication was very low in lean type 2 diabetics; 1% had coronary artery disease and 2% had cerebrovascular accident (Punyakrit *et al.*, 2011). In another Indian study also, ischemic heart disease was very low (2.7%) among lean type 2 diabetics, whereas it was 13.84% in normal weight 12% in over weight 23.07% in obese diabetics (Mukhyaprana *et al.*, 2004). Coronary heart disease prevalence was lower in lean group, but there was no difference in prevalence of stroke and peripheral arterial disease (Coleman *et al.*, 2014).

However, there was no significant difference in the prevalence of myocardial ischaemia or myocardial infarction between lean, ideal weight and obese T2DM from sex in the study by Mohan *et al.* (1997) The prevalence of peripheral vascular disease (PVD) was surprisingly higher among the lean patients of male sex compared to the obese group. However, the overall number of patients with PVD in the study was low.

6.8   Infections

Incidence of tuberculosis was very high in lean diabetics (26.6%) whereas tuberculosis was seen in 4% on of normal weight diabetics (Mukhyaprana *et al.*, 2004). Eight percent of patients had foot or systemic infections (Punyakrit *et al.*, 2011).

7 Response to treatment

In a randomized, single-blind, long-term study comparing unmeasured diet to exchange-type, calorically defined diet among lean T2DM the effect on fasting blood glucose, serum triglyceride, cholesterol, and weight was similar (Ikeda *et al.*, 1991).

Nearly 48% of the lean T2DM patients still responded to diet or oral hypoglycemic agents up to a mean duration of around 9 years (Mohan *et al.*, 1997). A higher percentage of lean (49%) versus obese (44%) patients required the use of insulin for glycemic control ($p = 0.001$) (Pontiroli *et al.*, 1992). In a Chinese study there were more subjects in the underweight group (41.3%) who were treated with insulin compared to normal weight (13.9%) and overweight (8.2%); $P < 0.001$ (Chan *et al.*, 2004).

Secondary oral hypoglycemic agent (OHA) failure was seen in 27% (Punyakrit *et al.*, 2011). Patients with secondary failure to sulphonylurea, similar to their responsive counterparts, failed to show insulin secretory response to intravenous glucose. But in comparison they have significantly reduced but not complete absence of insulin response to tolbutamide and glucagon. Amount of glucose metabolized and insulin sensitivity is also reduced in lean subjects (Pontiroli *et al.*, 1992).

8 Conclusion

A large chunk of type 2 diabetes patients are lean, the prevalence depending upon the population studied and the cut-off level used. There is a higher preponderance among males in contrast to female preponderance among obese. Most clamp studies show insulin secretory defect as the predominant defect in contrast to predominant insulin resistance in obese. Nearly half of these patients still respond to OHA even after a mean duration of around 10 years. Compared to obese type 2 diabetes they have a lesser prevalence of macrovascular complications.

References

Alberti, K.G., Zimmet, P., Shaw, J. (2006). *Metabolic syndrome — a new world-wide definition. A Consensus Statement from the International Diabetes Federation. Diabet Med. 2006. 23:469–80.*

Arnab, G. (2006). *Anthropometric, metabolic and dietary fatty acids profiles in lean and obese diabetic Asian Indian subjects. Asia Pac J Clin Nutr. 2006. 15(2):189–195.*

Arner, P., Pollare, T., Lithell, H. (1991). *Different aetiologies of type 2 (non-insulin-dependent) diabetes mellitus in obese and non-obese subjects. Diabetologia. 1991. 34(7):483–7.*

Banerji, M.A., Lebovitz, H.E. (1992). *Insulin action in black Americans with NIDDM. Diabetes Care. 1992. 15(10):1295–302.*

Bruno, G., De Salvia, A., Arcari, R. et al. (1999). *Clinical, immunological, and genetic heterogeneity of diabetes in an Italian population-based cohort of lean newly diagnosed patients aged 30–54 years. Piedmont Study Group for Diabetes Epidemiology. Diabetes Care. 1999. 22:50–5.*

Butler, A.E., Janson, J., Bonner-Weir, S., et al. (2003). *ß-Cell Deficit and Increased ß-Cell Apoptosis in Humans With Type 2 Diabetes. Diabetes. 2003. 52:102–10.*

Chan, W.B., Tong, P.C., Chow, C.C., et al. (2004). *The associations of body mass index, C-peptide and metabolic status in Chinese Type 2 diabetic patients. Diabet Med. 2004. 21(4):349–53.*

Chaudhary, P., Laloo, D., Salam, R. (2013). *Prevalence of lean type 2 diabetes mellitus in recently diagnosed type 2 diabetes mellitus patients. Indian J Endocr Metab. 2013. 17:S316–7.*

Coleman, N.J.J, Miernik, J., Philipson, L., et al. (2014). *Lean versus obese diabetes mellitus patients in the United States minority population. Journal of Diabetes and Its Complications. 2014. 28:500–5.*

Daousi, C., Casson, I.F., Gill, G.V. et al. (2006). *Prevalence of obesity in type 2 diabetes in secondary care: association with cardiovascular risk factors. Postgrad Med J. 2006. 82:280–4.*

Das, S., Bhoi, S.K., Baliarsinha, A.K., et al. (2007). *Autoimmunity, Insulin Resistance and Beta Cell Function in Subjects with Low Body Weight Type 2 Diabetes Mellitus. Metab Syndr Relat Disord. 2007. 5(2):136–41.*

Das, S., Samal, K.C., Baliarsinha, A.K., Tripathy BB. (1995). *Lean (underweight) NIDDM – peculiarities and differences in metabolic and hormonal status – A pilot study. JAPI. 1995. 43:339–42.*

DeFronzo, R.A. (2004). *Pathogenesis of type 2 diabetes mellitus. Med Clin North Am. 2004. 88: 787–835.*

Deurenberg-Yap, M., Schmidt, G., van Staveren, W.A., et al. (2000). *The paradox of low body mass index and high body fat percentage among Chinese, Malays and Indians in Singapore. Int J Obes Relat Metab Disord. 2000. 24: 1011–7.*

Eberhardt, M.S., Ogden, C. (2004). *Prevalence of overweight and obesity among adults with diagnosed diabetes – United states, 1998–1994 and 1999–2002. Morb Mortal Wkly Rep. 2004. 53:1066–8.*

Gallagher, A.M., Abraira, C., Henderson, W.G. (1984). *A Four-year Prospective Trial of Unmeasured Diet In Lean Diabetic Adults. Diabetes Care. 1984. 7:557–65.*

García-Estévez, D.A., Araújo-Vilar, D., Saavedra-González, A., et al. (2002). *Glucose metabolism in lean patients with mild type 2 diabetes mellitus: Evidence for insulin-sensitive and insulin-resistant variants. Metabolism. 2002. 51:1047–52.*

Garvey, W.T., Huecksteadt, T.P., Matthei, S., et al. (1988). *Role of glucose transporters in the cellular insulin resistance of the type II non-insulin dependent diabetes mellitus. J Clin Invest. 1988. 81:1528–36.*

Handberg, A., Vaag, A., Damsbo, P., et al. (1990). Expression of insulin regutatable glucose transporters in skeletal muscle from Type 2 (non-insulin-dependent) diabetic patients. Diabetologia. 1990. 33:625–27.

Ikeda, T., Ochi, H., et al. (1991). Serum lipid and apolipoprotein levels in non-hypertensive lean NIDDM patients. Journal of Internal Medicine. 1991. 230:131–4.

International Diabetes Institute. (2000). The Asia-Pacific perspective: Redefining obesity and its treatment. 2000. 15–21.

Iwasaki, N., Cox, N.J., Wang, Y.Q., et al. (2003) Mapping genes influencing type 2 diabetes risk and BMI in Japanese subjects. Diabetes. 2003. 52:209–13

Kadowaki, T., Sekikawa, A., Murata, K., et al. (2006). Japanese men have larger areas of visceral adipose tissue than Caucasian men in the same levels of waist circumference in a population-based study. Int J Obes (Lond). 2006. 30: 1163–5.

Kelly, D.E., Mokan, M., Mandarino, L.J. (1993). Metabolic pathways of glucose in skeletal muscle of lean NIDDM patients. Diabetes Care. 1993. 16(8):1158–66.

Lu, B., Yang, Y., Song, X., et al. (2006). An evaluation of the International Diabetes Federation definition of metabolic syndrome in Chinese patients older than 30 years and diagnosed with type 2 diabetes mellitus. Metabolism. 2006. 55(8):1088–96.

Mannucci, E., Alegiani, S.S., Monami, M., et al. (2004). Indexes of abdominal adiposity in patients with type 2 diabetes. J Endocrinol Invest. 2004. 27:535–40.

Mohan, V., Vijayaprabha, R., Rema, M., et al. (1997). Clinical profile of lean NIDDM in South India. Diabetes Research and Clinical Practice. 1997. 38:101–8.

Mukhyaprana, P.M., Vidyasagar, S., Shashikiran, U. (2004). Clinical profile of type 2 diabetes mellitus and body mass index- Is there any correlation. Calicut Medical Journal. 2004. 2(4):e3

National Heart, Lung, and Blood Institute. (1998). Expert Panel on the Identification, Evaluation, and Treatment of Overweight and Obesity in Adults. Clinical guidelines on the identification, evaluation, and treatment of overweight and obesity in adults: the evidence report. Obes Res. 1998. 6 (Suppl. 2):51S–209S.

Okamoto, K., Iwasaki, N., Doi, K., et al. (2012). Inhibition of glucose-stimulated insulin secretion by KCNJ15, a newly identified susceptibility gene for type 2 diabetes. Diabetes. 2012. 61:1734–41.

Okamoto, K., Iwasaki, N., Nishimura, C., et al. (2010). Identification of KCNJ15 as a susceptibility gene in Asian patients with type 2 diabetes mellitus. Am J Hum Genet. 2010. 86:54–64.

Pedersen, O., Bak, J.F., Andersen, P.H., Lund, S., et al. (1990). Evidence against altered expression of GLUT 1 or GLUT 4 in skeletal muscle of patients with obesity or NIDDM. Diabetes. 1990. 39:865–870.

Perry, J.R., Voight, B.F., Yengo, L., et al. (2012). Stratifying type 2 diabetes cases by BMI identifies genetic risk variants in LAMA1 and enrichment for risk variants in lean compared to obese cases. PLoS Genet. 2012. 8:e1002741.

Piatti, P.M., Monti, L.D., Davis, S.N., et al. (1996). Effects of an acute decrease in non-esterified fatty acid levels on muscle glucose utilization and forearm indirect calorimetry in lean NIDDM patients. Diabetologia. 1996. 39:103–12.

Pigon, J., Giacca, A., Ostenson, C.G., et al. (1996). Normal hepatic insulin sensitivity in lean, mild noninsulin-dependent diabetic patients. J Clin Endocrinol Metab, 1996. 81(10):3702–8.

Pontiroli, A.E., Caviezel, F., Alberetto, M., et al. (1992). Secondary failure of oral hypoglycemic agents in lean patients with type 2 diabetes mellitus: insulin sensitivity, insulin response to different stimuli, and the role of cyclic-AMP. Diabete Metab. 1992. 18(1):25–31.

Punyakrit, D.B., Salam, R., Lallan P., Thangjam P.S. (2011). Clinical and biochemical profile of lean type 2 diabetes mellitus. Indian J Endocr Metab. 2011. 15:S40–3.

Rattarasarn, C., Leelawattana, R., Soonthornpun, S., et al. (2003). Regional abdominal fat distribution in lean and obese Thai type 2 diabetic women: relationships with insulin sensitivity and cardiovascular risk factors. Metabolism. 2003. 52(11):1444–7.

Roder, M.E., Dinesen, B., Hartling, S.G., et al. (1999). Intact Proinsulin and Cell Function in Lean and Obese Subjects With and Without Type 2 Diabetes. Diabetes Care. 1999. 22:609–14.

Suraamornkul, S., Kwancharoen, R., Ovartlarnporn, M., et al. (2010). Insulin clamp-derived measurements of insulin sensitivity and insulin secretion in lean and obese Asian (Thai) type 2 diabetic patients. Metab Syndr Relat Disord 2010:8(2):113–18.

Takahara, M., Kaneto, H., Katakami, N., et al. (2011). Impaired suppression of endogenous glucose production in lean Japanese patients with type 2 diabetes mellitus. Diabetes Res Clin Pract. 2011. 93:e1–2.

Taniguchi, A., Fukushima, M., Sakai, M., et al. (2000). The role of the body mass index and triglyceride levels in identifying insulin-sensitive and insulin-resistant variants in Japanese non-insulin-dependent diabetic patients. Metabolism. 2000. 49(8):1001–5.

Thanabalasingham, G., Owen, K.R. (2011). Diagnosis and management of maturity onset diabetes of the young (MODY). BMJ. 2011. 343:d6044 doi: 10.1136/bmj.d6044.

Tripathy, B.B., Kar, B.C. (1965). Observations on clinical patterns of diabetes in India. Diabetes. 1965. 14:404–12.

Tsai, F.J., Yang, C.F., Chen, C.C., et al. (2010). A genome-wide association study identifies susceptibility variants for type 2 diabetes in Han Chinese. PLoS Genet. 2010. 6:e1000847. doi:10.1371/journal.pgen.1000847.

Unnikrishnan, A.G., Singh, S.K., Sanjeevi, C.B. (2004). Prevalence of GAD65 Antibodies in Lean Subjects with Type 2 Diabetes. Ann NY Acad Sci. 2004. 1037:118–21.

Vikram, N.K., Misra, A., Pandey, R.M., et al. (2003). Anthropometry and body composition in northern Asian Indian patients with type 2 diabetes: receiver operating characteristics (ROC) curve analysis of body mass index with percentage body fat as standard. Diabetes

Nutr Metab. 2003. 16:32–40.

Vogt, B., Miihlbacher, C., Carrascosa, J., et al. (1992). Subcellular distribution of GLUT 4 in the skeletal muscle of lean Type 2 (non-insulin-dependent) diabetic patients in the basal state. Diabetologia. 1992. 35:456–63.

Chapter 7

The Role of Dermcidin Isoform 2 in Different Conditions Predisposing to Acute Coronary Syndrome

Asru Kumar Sinha[1], Sarbashri Bank[1,2], Debipriya Banerjee[1], Suman Bhattacharya[1,2], Pradipta Jana[1,2], Rajeshwary Ghosh[1], Gannareddy V. Girish[1] & Gausal A. Khan[1]

1   Introduction

Environmentally induced stresses have been recognized to be involved in the pathogenesis of different life-threatening conditions that includes cancer (*Gaudet et al., 2013*), diabetes mellitus both type 1 and type 2 (Maritim *et al.*, 2003), hypertension (Briones & Touyz, 2010) and acute coronary syndromes (ACS) (Maxwell & Lip, 1997). However, it is only recently, an environmentally induced oxidative stress protein has been identified to be dermcidin isoform 2 (DCN-2) (Ghosh *et al.*, 2010). This protein of molecular weight 11kDa has been reported to be synthesized due to various stresses which includes hypoxia, tobacco smoke and alcohol consumption. These stresses have been related to the development of acute myocardial infarction (AMI), one of the most deadly thrombotic disorder and a major killer of the human race (Page *et al.*, 1971).

Diabetes mellitus (DM), an abnormal increase of blood glucose level in the circulation, is a major world-wide public health problem. The condition is classified as:

1. Type 1 diabetes mellitus (T1DM) where the systemic synthesis of insulin, an essential hormone for carbohydrate metabolism for energy transduction, was severely impaired (Pfeifer *et al.*, 1981) and,

[1] Department of Biochemistry, Sinha Institute of Medical Science & Technology, India
[2] Department of Biochemistry, Vidyasagar University, India

2. Type 2 diabetes mellitus (T2DM) where the system became resistant to the hy-poglycemic effect of the hormone (Bogardus, 1993).

Although the impaired insulin synthesis in the pancreatic β cells was originally believed to be solely responsible for production and secretion of insulin when stimulat-ed by glucose (Hughes *et al.*, 1992), more recently it has been reported that the extra pancreatic insulin synthesis (Kojima *et al.*, 2004) particularly in the hepatic cells in the liver was a major source of glucose induced insulin synthesis and secretion. Indeed the amounts of insulin synthesized in the liver could be more than 10 fold than that in the pancreas (Ghosh *et al.*, 2010). In this context it should be mentioned that the occurrence of DM either T1DM or T2DM almost always leads to atherosclerosis that is responsible to cause a pro-thrombotic condition leading to the development of acute coronary syn-drome (ACS) due to atherosclerotic plaque rupture on the coronary artery where the platelets formed micro-aggregates embedded in fibrin mass (thrombus) which in conse-quence obstructs normal blood circulation in the musculature of the heart and thus ini-tiating ACS (Colman & Walsh, 1987; Fuster *et al.*, 1996). The environmentally induced stress protein DCN-2 was found to be involved in the genesis of both type 1 and type 2 DM leading to atherosclerosis. Thus DCN-2 may not only pre-dispose system to athero-sclerosis but may actually be involved in ACS (Ghosh *et al.*, 2011).

The environmentally induced stress protein might be involved in the pathogene-sis of AMI. AMI is developed due to thrombosis in the pericardium (Carvalho *et al.*, 1988), and that might extend to both left and right ventricle, usually cause cardiac cell death that appear as patchy dark spots on the heart surface. It has been reported by many investigators that the use of aspirin, through its ability to inhibit platelet aggrega-tion not only reduce the occurrence of death in ACS, but the compound has been re-ported to improve all acute syndromes associated with the condition (Pollack *et al.*, 1995). Unfortunately, however, aspirin has been reported to fail to inhibit platelet ag-gregation in AMI. Neither the mechanism of the resistance of the platelets to the inhibi-tory effect of aspirin in AMI nor the way to restore the sensitivity of the platelets to the aspirin effect that could be beneficial in AMI was until recently available. We have re-cently reported that the appearance of DCN-2 in the circulation in AMI, imparted the resistance of the AMI platelets to the inhibitory effect of aspirin (Bank *et al.*, 2014, Scien-tific Reports).

It is generally believed that high altitude illness (HAI) is a cluster of syndromes leading to life threatening condition of pro-thrombotic disease due to the development of ACS where the decent to sea level from high altitude condition usually produced lit-tle or no effect on the ensuing ACS. As such, persons stationed at high altitude are par-ticularly vulnerable to an attack of ACS. Unfortunately, however, neither the mecha-nism of the development of ACS due to prothrombotic condition, nor any diagnosis for the occurrence of prothrombotic condition, which could be used as a warning to stave off the ominous event that may precipitate ACS has yet been identified. Investigations was carried out on the effect of various altitude heights on the plasma DCN-2 level, that it could be of useful in the diagnosis of prothrombotic condition at high altitude. It was found that the appearance of DCN-2 in high altitude actually precipitated AMI (Bank *et al.*, 2014, Clinical Laboratory).

The death rate due to the occurrence of ACS or AMI in subjects with breast cancer is reported to be significantly higher than that in general female population at large. In this context, it has been reported before that while the death due to ACS or AMI in female population was 34%, the occurrence of breast cancer in the victims was found to increase the incidences of death due to ACS or AMI by ~50% (Darby *et al.*, 2013). The role of DCN-2 in development of ACS in patients with breast cancer was investigated and reported in the article.

Finally, although cholesterol is reported to be a risk factor for ACS (Libby, 2005), no mechanism for increased ACS due to hypercholesterolemia is known. It was found that DCN-2, a double edged risk factor for both DM and hypertension could be involved in the increased occurrences of atherosclerosis in hypercholesterolemia. As such, DCN-2 could be determined as a global mediator of atherosclerosis.

In this chapter, a brief and general view of the involvement of DCN-2 in the pathogenic development of different conditions leading to ACS has been described herein.

2   Material and Methods

2.1   Ethical Clearance

Wherever appropriate the protocol described was approved by the Internal Review Board, Sinha Institute of Medical Science and Technology, Calcutta. All participants were asked to sign informed consent form. This study also used normal white Swiss albino mice (Mus musculus) and adult New Zealand rabbit. Appropriate permission was obtained from the IRB.

2.2   Selection of AMI Patients

All patients ($n = 29$) between ages of 49 and 61 (median age 54 years) were admitted to the Intensive Care Unit of the Calcutta Medical College and Hospital, Kolkata. These patients met the following criteria of AMI: they had chest pain characteristic of myocardial ischemia for 30 mins or more and the electrocardiogram (ECG) showed ST segment elevation of at least two leads in the ECG reflecting a single myocardial region. The confirmation of the condition was determined by plasma troponin I. The sampling of blood was made within 6 h of the onset of the anginal attack before any therapy for the condition was initiated. Only those AMI patients who refused to ingest aspirin due to personal/religious beliefs served as "controls" when necessary.

2.2.1   Exclusion Criteria

(1) Patients with the history of diabetes mellitus, (2) showing the presence of bundle branch block or left ventricular hypertrophy in the ECG (3) or suffering from any severe infection, (4) took aspirin at least within 2 weeks, (5) hospitalized for any condition

within two months, and (6) took any cardiac medication including any antihypertensive drug within last 21 days were excluded from the study.

2.3   Collection of Blood

Blood samples (2–5mL), obtained from the participants by venipuncture by using 19-gauge siliconized needles, were collected in plastic vials and anticoagulated by gently mixing 9 vol of the blood with 1 vol of 0.13mM sodium citrate (Karmohapatra *et al.*, 2003). The cell-free plasma (CFP) was prepared by centrifuging the blood sample from the participants at 30,000 g for 30 min at 0∘C.

2.4   Preparation of DCN-2

DCN-2 was prepared from the blood of the subjects suffering from ACS by using SDS-Poly acryl amide gel electrophoresis as described before in detail (Ghosh *et al.*, 2011).

2.5   Assay of DCN-2

The plasma DCN-2 was determined by Enzyme Linked Immunosorbent Assay (ELISA) using antibody raised against electrophoretically purified DCN-2 as the antigen in New Zealand white rabbit that has been described in detail before (Ghosh *et al.*, 2011).

2.6   Assay on the Effect of DCN-2 on Hypertension and DM

All the assays regarding the effects of DCN-2 on hypertension both in humans (Ghosh *et al.*, 2014, Cardiology Research and Practice) and in animal model (Ghosh *et al.*, 2012, Thrombosis) and T1DM in human model (Ghosh *et al.*, 2010, Ghosh *et al.*, 2012, International Journal of Biomedical Science, Ghosh *et al.*, 2011) and in animal model (Ghosh *et al.*, 2012, Experimental Clinical Endocrinology Diabetes, Bhattacharya *et al.*, 2013) and T2DM in animal model (Ghosh *et al.*, 2014, Cardiology Research and Practice) has been described before.

2.7   Effect of DCN-2 on Aggregation of Platelets, HAI, AMI

Assays related to DCN-2 as an effective platelet aggregating agent (Ghosh *et al.*, 2014, Cardiology Research and Parctice), HAI [Bank *et al.*, 2014, Clinical Laboratory] and in AMI [Bank *et al.*, 2014, Scientific Reports] has been described before.

2.8   Selection of Subjects with Hypercholesterolemia

The blood samples were collected from the subjects with different degree of hypercholesterolemia ranging from 140mg cholesterol/dL of cholesterol (desirable) to 250mg cholesterol/dL (abnormally high). As the cholesterol levels in the participating subjects were intrinsically variable, the patients were divided into groups where each group consists of five subjects (total = 70) whose cholesterol level differs by 10mg/dl either way.

2.9 Effect of Hypercholesterolemia on the Synthesis of Dermcidin mRNA

Leukocyte suspension was prepared from the venous blood which was withdrawn by using 19-gauge siliconized needle and was collected in plastic vial. The blood sample was anticoagulated by adding 1vol of sodium citrate to 9vol of blood as described before (Karmohapatra et al., 2003). Leukocytes were isolated from the buffy coat and purified by ficoll histopaque gradient (Klock & Bainton, 1976). The leukocyte preparation was suspended in Tyrode's buffer pH 7.4 and was used as soon as possible.

Typically, the leukocytes suspension in Tyrode's buffer pH 7.4, was treated with cholesterol and pure lecithin in the ratio 1:2, for 2h 30min at 37^{0}C, the nucleic acids containing mRNA for DCN-2 were extracted by Trizol method (Ganguly et al., 2013), the nucleic acid extract was treated with the mixture of 1nM of all 20 different amino acids and 1.0μM ATP and the mRNA was translated by using plant leaf ribosomal particles (Ganguly et al., 2013). The synthesized proteins that also contained DCN-2 was determined by ELISA as described above.

In vitro experiments were performed to determine the effect of DCN-2 in goat artery endothelial cells incubated with 1:2 ratio of cholesterol and lecithin for 2h 30min at 37^{0}C.

2.10 Selection of Breast Cancer Patients

Only female breast cancer patients 25 to 55 years of age (n = 1140) participated in the study. The breast cancer was diagnosed by mammogram followed by biopsy and was categorized by TNM classification at presentation. Those patients who were undergoing therapies including chemotherapy, radiation and even surgery was not included in the study. These volunteers were given appropriate legal counseling in the presence of their family members and legal counselors. All selected volunteers were asked to obtain judicial affidavit from the court of law and signed informed consent form. They were also advised to discontinue aspirin any time they wanted and they were at liberty to begin use of any therapy including chemotherapy, radiation or surgery for their condition without any consent from the investigators at any time.

2.11 In Vitro Translation of DCN-2 Synthesis in Leukocytes by Ethanol

Typically, the leukocytes suspension in Tyrode's buffer pH 7.4, was treated with different amounts of ethanol, as described above. The synthesized proteins that also contained DCN-2 was determined by ELISA as described above.

2.12   Preparation of Cell Free Supernatant from the Disrupted Platelet Mass

The PRP was prepared from a single donor and centrifuged at 10,000g for 30min at 0°C. The platelet mass was resuspended in 1.0ml of Tyrode's buffer pH7.4 and disrupted by freezing and thawing in liquid N_2. The disrupted mass was centrifuged at 30,000g, for 30min at 0°C. The supernatant was collected and used as the source of NOS.

2.13   Lineweaver-Burk Plot of the Nitric Oxide Synthase (NOS) Activity of the Supernatant from the Disrupted Platelet Mass

Typically 0.2mL of the supernatant of the disrupted platelet mass was treated with 2.0mM $CaCl_2$ in the presence or absence of 2.0μM ADP and different amounts of *l*-arginine (substrate of NOS) in a total volume of 1.0mL in Tyrode's buffer pH7.4 and incubated for 5min at 37°C. The formation of NO in the supernatant was determined by methemoglobin method as described below.

2.14   Determination of NO

NO was determined by methemoglobin method as described before (Jia *et al.*, 1996, Sinha *et al.*, 1999). The amounts of NO formed was verified by independent chemiluminescence method (Cox & Frank, 1982).

2.15   Determination of Blood Glucose Level

The blood glucose level was determined by a glucometer (Behringer).

2.16   Determination of Blood Pressure Levels

The systolic and diastolic blood pressures were measured by using mercury sphygmomanometer.

3   Results

3.1   The role of DCN-2 in the Development of T1DMB in Hepatic Insulin Synthesis

We have reported before that the hepatic synthesis of insulin remained functional even when the pancreatic synthesis of the hormone was severely impaired as in the case of T1DM (Ghosh *et al.*, 2010). As such, the issue remains "why there should be any T1DM if the glucose was capable of stimulating and secreting bio-active insulin in the hepatocytes in the liver?". It was found that for the hepatic synthesis of insulin in the presence of glucose as well as the synthesis of NO is critically important (Ghosh *et al.*, 2010). As

DCN-2 was found to be present in the liver and the protein was a potent inhibitor of nitric oxide synthases (Ghosh *et al.*, 2010), the glucose induced hepatic synthesis and secretion of insulin in the hepatic cells was nullified in the absence of NO synthesis inhibited by DCN-2 (Ghosh *et al.*, 2010). However, the inhibitory effect of DCN-2 could be nullified by increasing systemic NO synthesis either by applying sodium nitroprusside patch on the skin or by oral administration of aspirin (Ghosh *et al.*, 2011) that effectively controlled the hyperglycemia in alloxan induced T1DM in animal model (Ghosh *et al.*, 2012, Experimental Clinical & Endocrinology Diabetes) and in T1DMB in humans (Ghosh *et al.*, 2012, International Journal of Biomedical Science) through the hepatic synthesis of insulin without the use of any external insulin.

Similar results were also obtained by the neutralization of the DCN-2 effect on the inhibition of insulin in hepatic cells by stimulating nitric oxide synthase by using nM quantity of estrogen or particularly progesterone which are reported before to be potent activators of NOS synthase (Bhattacharya *et al.*, 2014).

We have reported before that at least 65% of the T1DM patients in India might be categorized as T1DMB and the plasma concentration of DCN-2 in these subjects were >124nM that contrasted the plasma DCN-2 of 15nM in non-diabetic age and sex matched volunteers (Ghosh *et al.*, 2011). The increase of plasma DCN-2 was highly correlated to the hyperglycemia in these subjects (Ghosh *et al.*, 2011).

3.2   The Role of DCN-2 in the Synthesis of Insulin in the Hepatic Cells and in the Pancreatic Islets of Langerhans

We have recently reported the existence of a glucose activated nitric oxide synthase (GANOS) in the liver. This enzyme (GANOS) was found to have critically important role in glucose activated NO synthesis in the production of insulin in the hepatic cells, not only in the glucose induced synthesis in the liver, but also in the secretion of insulin through the conversion of pro-insulin to bioactive insulin in the hepatic cells (Bhattacharya *et al.*, 2013) by the activation of plasminogen in the circulation to plasmin by glucose induced nitric oxide synthase (GANOS). DCN-2 was reported to be a potent inhibitor of all known forms of nitric oxide synthases through its ability to be a competitive inhibitor of *l*-arginine, only known substrate for all forms of NO synthases. The liver GANOS was found to be very sensitive to the inhibitory effect of DCN-2, and as a result, the hepatic synthesis of insulin by DCN-2 resulted in the severe impairment of hepatic insulin synthesis leading to overt T1DMB (Bhattacharya *et al.*, 2013) (Figure 1).

3.3   The Effect of Injection of DCN-2 in the Mice Circulation in the Synthesis of Insulin and on the Hyperglycemia

As discussed above, the cause for the development of T1DM remains obscure. However, when 0.2 μM dermcidin was injected in the tail vein of the test animals and the blood glucose and insulin levels were determined at different time intervals. The blood glucose level which was 98 ± 2.45mg/dL before the injection of dermcidin was found to be elevated to 350 ± 10.2 mg/dL at 160min after the injection of the stress-induced protein

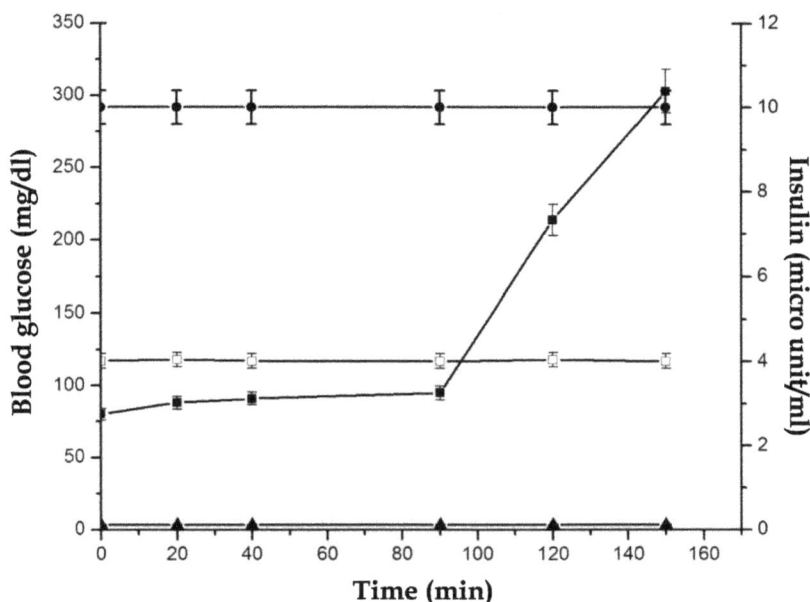

Figure 1: The effect of DCN-2 on the development of T1DM like condition in mice.

with concomitant decrease of the plasma insulin level from 35.56 ± 2.42 μunits/ml to 4.56 ± 0.018 μunits/ml after the injection. Further studies demonstrated that the blood glucose level of 350 ± 0.2 mg/dL as well as the insulin level of 4.56 ± 0.018 μunits/dL remained nearly unchanged for the next 120mins. However, after 24 h of dermcidin injection, both blood glucose levels and insulin levels were found to return to their normal ranges.

3.4   The effect of DCN-2 on the Development of T2DM in Mice Model

As stated above, currently there is no mechanism known for the development of T2DM (Rathsman *et al.*, 2012). Indeed, the effect of T2DM on the increased abdominal obesity has been recently confusingly claimed to be the cause of T2DM (Pal D., *et al.* 2012). On the other hand, as described below, it was found that the injection of 0.24µM DCN-2 in the circulation of adult mice caused acute increase of the blood glucose level to 320mg/dl from the basal 60mg/dl. However, it was also noted that the plasma insulin level simultaneously increased to 35µunits/ml from 10-15µunits of insulin/ml indicating that despite the glucose induced increased synthesis of insulin, the hypoglycemic hormone failed to control hyperglycemia (Figure 2), thus suggesting the development of systemic insulin resistance, a hallmark of T2DM. Furthermore, it was also found that insulin resistance could be overcome by injecting 25µunits of insulin in the system suggesting that the amount of insulin produced by the glucose in the animal was not ade-

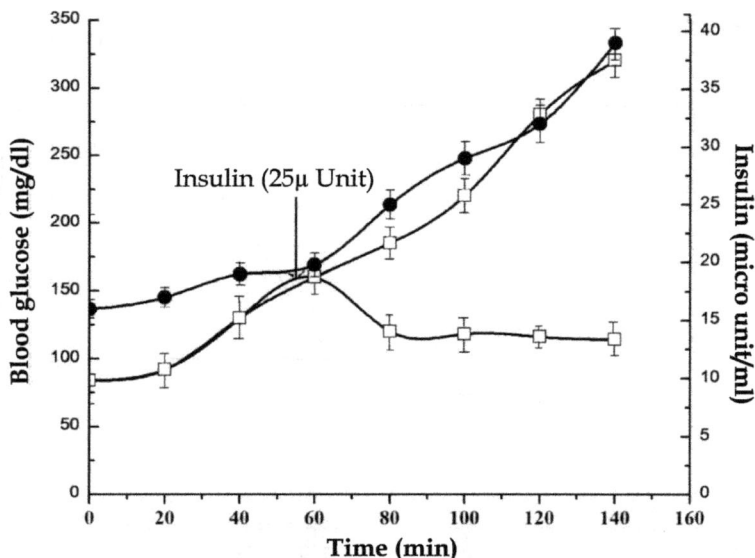

Figure 2: The effects of DCN-2 on the blood glucose and plasma insulin level in adult mice.

quate to control hyperglycemia, and the injection of external insulin that made up for the inadequate availability of the systemic insulin "corrected" the hyperglycemia, a typical pathologic event in T2DM in man where the glucose induced insulin synthesis and release were impaired (Bogardus, 1993). T2DM could be also induced by feeding aqueous tobacco leaf extract or pure nicotine which was found to increase plasma DCN-2 level (Ghosh *et al.*, 2014, Cardiology Research & Practice).

Adult mice (25–30gm) fed ad-libitum were injected with 0.24 µM DCN-2 in the circulation. At different times as indicated, after the injection of DCN-2, both the blood glucose and plasma insulin levels were determined. In control experiments, equal volume of 0.9% NaCl (vehicle for DCN-2) was used. Results shown are mean ± S.D. of 10 different animals. The solid circles (●) show the plasma insulin level. The open squares (□) represent the blood glucose level. In the same experiment, 25µunits of insulin/DCN-2 treated mice was injected at 50min in these mice (as instructed by ↓) and the blood glucose and plasma insulin levels were determined after the injection of the external insulin at different times as indicated.

3.5   The role of DCN-2 on the Increase of Arterial Blood Pressure in Hypertensive Human Subjects

We have reported before that in human hypertensive patients, the increased presence of DCN-2 in the plasma could be demonstrated, and the oral administration of acetyl salicylic acid (aspirin) normalized the increased plasma DCN-2 levels from 95nM to 15nM (normal concentration of DCN-2 in the patients suffering from ACS) within 3h of ingestion of the compound. In hypertensive subjects, the oral administration of aspirin decreased the systolic pressure from 165mm of Hg to 125mm of Hg with the simultaneous decrease of diastolic pressure from 95mm of Hg to 80mm of Hg and with decrease of the intensity of the DCN-2 band in the SDS-polyacrylamide gel, suggesting that in humans the aspirin induced decrease of the plasma DCN-2 level controlled the increase of both systolic and diastolic pressure (Ghosh *et al.*, 2014, Cardiology Research & Practice). The effect of injection of DCN-2 in rabbits increased the systolic pressure from 155 ± 4.78mm of Hg to 200 ± 10mm of Hg with simultaneous increase of diastolic pressure of 57.5 ± 8.66mm Hg to 125 ± 5.77mmHg after 2 h of the injection (Ghosh *et al.*, 2012, Thrombosis).

These results as described above strongly suggest that DCN-2 was a potent atherosclerotic risk factor through its ability to simultaneously cause both T1DMB and hypertension both in humans and in the animal model. As DM and hypertension are reported to be the two major risk factors for atherosclerosis leading to ACS, the environmentally induced stress protein DCN-2 could play a critically important role in the development of atherosclerosis.

3.6   The Role of DCN-2 as a Potent Cycloxygenase Activator in Platelets

We have reported before that DCN-2 was a potent platelet aggregating agent as a cycloxygenase activator similar to that of the well known human platelet aggregating agent ADP (Ghosh *et al.*, 2014, Cardiology Research & Practice). However, it was estimated that DCN-2 was at least 40-fold more effective platelet aggregating agent when compared to that of ADP.

3.7   The Effect of DCN-2 in the Development of ACS/AMI in High Altitude Illness

Personnel stationed in high altitude areas, persons travelling in airplane for prolonged period of time or sportsmen engaged in their sporting activities in high altitude areas are sometime reported to develop high altitude illness (Hackett & Roach, 2001). Although these high altitude illnesses are temporary conditions in nature, the high altitude induced illness usually and rapidly subsides when brought to the ground level. However, high altitude illness may also precipitate ACS/AMI.

Although few bureaucratic health official in certain countries, due to their lack of understanding on the pathogenesis of the prothrombotic condition leading to ACS or AMI, sometime claimed that high altitude illness is a "geographical disease". We have recently reported that both ACS or AMI in the high altitude illness was due to the increase of DCN-2 in the circulation which was reported to help ACS to convert to dangerous AMI (Bank *et al.*, 2014, Scientific Reports) please see below and when that happened, neither aspirin improve the condition nor bringing the victim at ground level can help them. And, as a result, the victims may die particularly due to AMI due to high altitude illness (Bank *et al.*, 2014, Clinical Laboratory).

3.8   The Role of DCN-2 as the Cause of Severe Cardiac Pain in ACS and AMI

The development of characteristic cardiac pain in ACS and the development of even more severe cardiac pain in AMI (Everts *et al.*, 1996) can be defined as the "hallmark" of these conditions in humans.

Unfortunately, however no acceptable mechanism of the severe cardiac pain in these conditions was available. We, recently have demonstrated, that the lack of systemic NO level was probably the cause of the cardiac pain in that the basal NO level in the plasma of AMI patients was found to reduce to undetectable ranges (~0nmol/ml) from 4nM in normal volunteers across the ethnic and geographical barriers (Ghosh *et al.*, 2014, PloS ONE). The lack of systemic NO level was related to the increase of DCN-2 level in these conditions where the level of DCN-2 was 4 to 40 fold higher in AMI than that in ACS which inhibited the systemic synthesis of NO induced by all known forms of NOS (Ghosh *et al.*, 2014, PloS ONE).

That the systemic increase of NO could rapidly control the cardiac pain in these conditions by using "nitro" compounds supported the role of NO in the control of cardiac pain in these conditions (Ghosh *et al.*, 2014, PloS ONE). Both aspirin (Karmohapatra *et al.*, 2007) and insulin (Bhattacharya *et al.*, 2001) through their ability to increase systemic NO level also reported to control the cardiac pain in ACS and AMI (Ghosh *et al.*, 2014, PloS ONE).

3.9   The Acute Effect of DCN-2 in the Nullification of the Aspirin Induced Inhibition of Platelet Aggregation in Acute Myocardial Infarction

Although the development of thrombosis in the arteries of the heart leads to ACS (Colman *et al.*, 1987; Fuster *et al.*, 1996), sometimes thrombosis interrupts the normal blood circulation in the heart. And, as a result of the blockage of blood circulation in the pericardium leads to the death of cardiac cells that caused acute myocardial infarction (AMI). The platelets from AMI unexplainably however became resistant to the inhibition of aggregation by aspirin, and as such the prevention of recurrences of AMI remains very difficult due to lack of suitable and effective inhibitor of platelet aggregation similar to that produced by aspirin.

We have recently reported that the binding of DCN-2 on its receptor sites on the platelet membrane in AMI, where the plasma DCN-2 level increased by 40 folds more than normal and more than 5 folds compared to ACS, resulted in the nullification of the inhibitory effect of aspirin (Bank *et al.*, 2014, Scientific Reports). However, the platelet bound DCN-2 could be removed by increasing NO synthesis in the platelets that rendered the platelets from AMI to become "supertensive" to the inhibitory effect of aspirin in that the platelets from AMI subject could be inhibited (100%) by only 25µM aspirin.

3.10   Association of DCN-2 in Hypercholesterolemia

Hypercholesterolemia, also known as dyslipidemia, is a well known risk factor for ACS (Libby, 2005). Unfortunately however, the increased occurrence of ACS in hypercholesterolemia remains hypothetical. Furthermore, whether hypercholesterolemia may actually increase the platelet aggregation to increase thrombosis in the coronary artery leading to increased occurrence of ACS remains debatable.

The determination of the plasma DCN-2 level in hypercholesterolemia subjects (ranging from 140mg/dl to 270mg cholesterol/dL) demonstrated, that while the DCN-2 level in the age and sex matched normal volunteers had ~15nM DCN-2, the atherosclerotic risk factor was increased to 130nM of DCN-2 ($n = 70$) in hypercholesterolemic subjects, which was found to be related to the increase of the plasma cholesterol level from 140 to 260mg cholesterol/dL in the participating hypercholesterolemic patients (Figure 3).

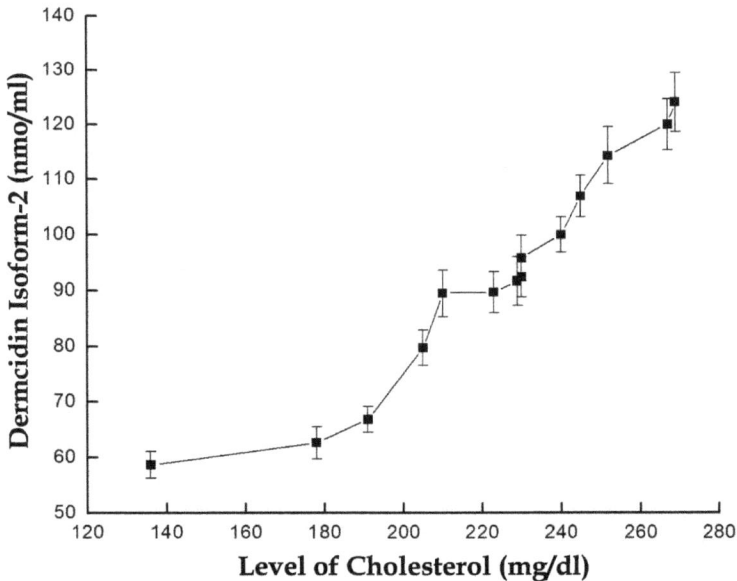

Figure 3: The effect of increased cholesterol level in hypercholesterolemia on the increase of plasma DCN-2 level.

As described in Methods and Materials, the mean of the cholesterol level of each group was used as shown in the x-axis of the figure. Results shown are mean ± S.D. as indicated above.

Furthermore, the treatment of goat carotid artery endothelial cells suspension in Tyrode's buffer in the presence of cholesterol and pure lecithin (1:2) as described in materials and methods resulted in the increased synthesis of DCN-2 from the control (Lecithin only) 132pmol/ml to 190pmol/ml ($p < 0.0005$, $n = 50$).

3.11   The Role of DCN-2 in Breast Cancer in the Development of ACS in Female Breast Cancer Patients

The development of breast cancer in the female subjects has been reported to result in the increased incidences of ACS (Darby *et al.*, 2013). In a pilot study, when the level of DCN-2 in female breast cancer patients was determined, it was found that the level of DCN-2 increased from 15.50 ± 0.64nM to 36.75 ± 0.85nM ($p < 0.001$) (Figure 4). As aspirin has been reported to neutralize the synthesis of DCN-2, in another study 1140 patients were asked to ingest 14mg aspirin/70 kg body weight for 2years (The study was regis-tered with the Clinical Trial Registration India (CTRI), trail registration no: CTRI/2014/12/ 005235), it was found that the rate of death due to ACS or AMI in breast cancer patients who had received 14mg of aspirin/70Kg body weight for 2years was 10.43% that contrasted the death rate (50%) who didn't receive aspirin. Z-test analysis between the groups were performed where the calculated Z value of the death rate due to ACS or AMI between the normal population and the breast cancer patients who re-ceived aspirin was 17.36 which was greater than the critical two-tailed z value 2.17. Al-so, the z-value of the death rates due to ACS or AMI between the breast cancer patients not receiving aspirin and the breast cancer patients using aspirin was 27.34 which was again greater than the critical two-tailed z-value 2.33. The P-value for the two-tailed test in all the cases was found to be 0 which was less than the alpha value of 0.5 (i.e. $P < 0.5$). Thus Z-test analysis of the death rate due to ACS or AMI in normal, breast cancer pa-tients and the breast cancer patients who received aspirin demonstrated that the use of aspirin could be useful for the prevention of death rate due to ACS or AMI in female breast cancer patients.

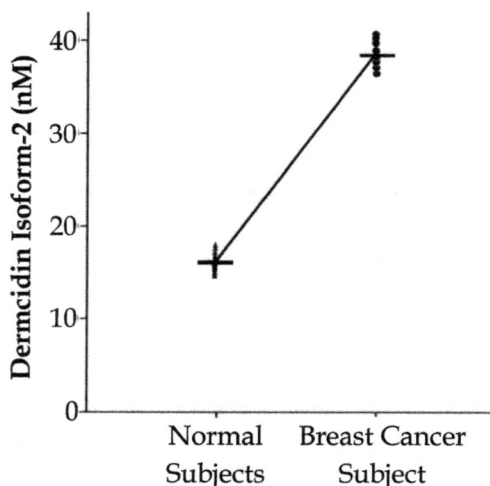

Figure 4: Quantitation of DCN-2 in plasma in breast cancer subjects and in age matched normal female volunteers.

Citrated blood was collected from breast cancer volunteers and normal female volunteers and the plasma DCN-2 was determined by ELISA using antibody raised against electrophoretically pure DCN-2 as the antigen. The values shown are represented as mean ± S.D. of twenty eight different breast cancer subjects and equal number of age matched normal female volunteers. The significance of the increase of plasma DCN-2 level was determined by Student's t-test where $p < 0.01$. Symbol (●) represents breast cancer volunteers and symbol (▲) represents normal volunteers.

4   Discussion

The development of atherosclerotic plaque in the coronary artery that resulted in the prothrombotic condition is reported to be the leading cause for the development of ACS in humans (Colman *et al.*, 1987; Fuster *et al.*, 1996) while atherosclerosis itself known to be a natural condition, mechanism for the condition remains obscure. Perhaps, more importantly, atherosclerosis once developed on the coronary artery; there is no known non-invasive way to remove the plaque from the wall of the coronary artery. In this context, it must be mentioned here that extensive trial with aspirin in human volunteers has demonstrated that this compound was capable of reducing the incidences of ACS, a major killer disease of the human race (Pollack, 1995). The mechanism of aspirin effect on the reduction of the occurrences of ACS has been reported to be due to the inhibition of platelet aggregation (Pollack, 1995).

At present, only known way to prevent atherosclerosis is to control DM (both T1DM and T2DM) and hypertension (Sowers *et al.*, 2001). These two independent risk factors are however were capable of influencing each other, and considered to be the two major risk factors for atherosclerosis (Kosiborod, 2008; Goldberg *et al.*, 2007; Sowers *et al.*, 2001). Even dyslipidemia including hypercholesterolemia that can cause atherosclerosis and deregulated thrombolysis all are reported to be the consequences of T2DM (Goldberg, 2001). And as such, the inhibition of platelet aggregation by aspirin through the inhibition of cycloxygenase cannot control either hypertension or diabetes mellitus (either type 1 or type 2). The effect of aspirin has been reported to be due to the activation of a constitutive form nitric oxide synthase that has been purified to homogeneity (Karmohapatra *et al.*, 2007). Nitric oxide thus formed was capable of neutralizing the effect of DCN-2 as a atherosclerotic risk factor through its ability to control both hypertension (Ghosh *et al.*, 2014, Cardiology Research and Practice) and diabetes mellitus (Ghosh *et al.*, 2012, ECED; Ghosh *et al.*, 2012, International Journal of Biomedical Science).

Although hypercholesterolemia is decidedly a potent risk factor for ACS, its mechanism of action remains hypothetical and even enigmatic, and the molecule itself is an essential component of cell membrane as well as a precursor molecule of all steroids. As described above, the increase of plasma cholesterol that led to the increased synthesis of DCN-2 in the endothelial cells strongly suggested, that the increase of plasma cholesterol level similar to other environmentally induced risk factor for atherosclerosis, led to the increased synthesis of DCN-2, a potent double edged atherosclerotic risk factor (Ghosh *et al.*, 2012, Thrombosis). Interestingly, in a preliminary study, it was found that the presence of aspirin in the reaction mixture inhibited the synthesis of DCN-2 through its ability to stimulate NO synthesis in the endothelial cells [unpublished], suggesting possible use of aspirin in hypercholesterolemia to control increased DCN-2 synthesis and consequently atherosclerosis.

DCN-2, an environmentally induced stress protein which was found to be simultaneously an inducer of both T1DM as well as T2DM (Ghosh *et al.*, 2012, Thrombosis; Ghosh *et al.*, 2014, Cardiology Research & Practice) was also found to be associated with hypertension T2DM (Ghosh *et al.*, 2012, Thrombosis; Ghosh *et al.*, 2014, Cardiology Research & Practice), and as such, the protein could be an all-round atherosclerotic risk factor. The plasma level of this protein was found to be increased in different and sometimes unrelated diseases (including DM, hypertension, hypercholesterolemia or even breast cancer) all of which are previously demonstrated to cause ACS in the victims through increased atherosclerosis. It should be mentioned here, that the increase of DCN-2 level in the reaction mixture as in the case of hypercholesterolemia as described above or in the cases of different environmentally induced stresses including hypoxia, nicotine aqueous extract of the tobacco leaf or alcohol (Ghosh *et al.*, 2014, Cardiology Research & Practice), was not due to the release of preformed DCN-2 from the cells in the mixture, but was related to the synthesis of DCN-2 in each case, was demonstrated to be actual synthesis of the protein by *in vitro* mRNA translation (Ghosh *et al.*, 2014, Cardiology Research & Practice) due to appropriate gene expression.

5   Conclusion

The protein DCN-2 was found to be involved in the development of T1DM, T2DM, hypertension, AMI, high altitude illness, hypercholesterolemia and ACS in breast cancer, thus indicating all round detrimental role of DCN-2 in ACS in both human and animal model. Interestingly, the use of aspirin has shown to inhibit systemic DCN-2 synthesis through the stimulation of mRNA by the activation of aspirin activated nitric oxide synthase leading to the synthesis of NO.

References

Bank, S., Ghosh, R., Jana, P., Bhattacharya, S. & Sinha, A.K. (2014). *The Diagnosis of High Altitude Illness by the Determination of Plasma Dermcidin Isoform 2 Levels by Enzyme Linked Immunosorbent Assay. Clinical Laboratory*, 60, doi: 10.7754/Clin.Lab.2013.130409.

Bank; S., Jana, P., Maiti, S., Guha, S. & Sinha, A.K. (2014). *Dermcidin isoform-2 induced nullification of the effect of acetyl salicylic acid in platelet aggregation in acute myocardial infarction. Scientific Reports*, 4,5804.

Bhattacharya, S., Basuray, S., Chakroborty, S. & Sinha, A.K. (2001). *Purification and properties of insulin activated nitric oxide synthase from human red cell membrane. Archives of*

Physiology & Biochemistry, 109,441–449.

Bhattacharya, S., Ghosh, R., Maiti, S., Khan, G.A. & Sinha, A.K. (2013). *The Activation by Glucose of Liver Membrane Nitric Oxide Synthase in the Synthesis and Translocation of Glucose transporter-4 in the Production of Insulin in the Mice Hepatocytes. PLoS ONE, 8(12),e81935.*

Bhattacharya, S., Bank, S., Maiti, S. & Sinha, A.K. (2014). *The Control of Hyperglycemia by Estriol and Progesterone in Alloxan induced Type I Diabetes Mellitus Mice Model through Hepatic Insulin Synthesis. International Journal of Biomedical Sciences, 10(1),8–15.*

Bogardus, C. (1993). *Insulin resistance in the pathogenesis of NIDDM in Pima Indians. Diabetes Care, 16,228–231.*

Briones, M. & Touyz, R.M. (2010). *Oxidative stress and hypertension: current concepts. Current Hypertension Reports,12(2),135–142.*

Carvalho De Sousa, J., Azevedo, J., Soria, C., Barros, F., Ribeiro, C., Parreira, F. & Caen, J.P. (1988). *Factor VII hyperactivity in acute myocardial thrombosis. A relation to the coagulation activation. Thrombosis Research,15,165–73.*

Colman, R.W. & Walsh, P.N. (1987). *Haemostasis and thrombosis. J.B. Lippincott, Philadelphia, P.A.*

Cox, R.D. & Frank, C.W. (1982). *Determination of nitrate and nitrite in blood and urine by chemiluminescence. Journal of Analytical Toxicology, 6,148–152.*

Darby, S.C., Ewertz, M., McGale, P., Bennet, A.M., Blom-Goldman, U., Brønnum, D., Correa, C., Cutter, D., Gagliardi, G., Gigante, B., Jensen, M.B., Nisbet, A., Peto, R., Rahimi, K. & Taylor, C. (2013). *Risk of ischemic heart disease in women after radiotherapy for breast cancer. New England Journal of Medicine, 368,987–998.*

Everts, B., Karlson, B.W., Währborg, P., Hedner, T. & Herlitz, J. (1996). *Localization of pain in suspected acute myocardial infarction in relation to final diagnosis, age and sex, and site and type of infarction. Heart & Lung: The Journal of Acute and Critical Care, 25(6),430–437.*

Fuster, V., Badimon, J., Chesebro, J.H. & Fallon, J.T. (1996). *Plaque rupture, thrombosis, and therapeutic implications. Haemostasis, 26,269–284.*

Ganguly, B.K., Bhattacharyya, M., Halder, U.C., Jana, P. & Sinha, A.K. (2012). *The Role of Neutrophil Estrogen Receptor Status on Maspin Synthesis via Nitric Oxide Production in Human Breast Cancer. Journal of Breast Cancer, 15,181–188.*

Gaudet, M.M., Gapstur, S.M., Sun, J., Diver, W.R., Hannan, L.M. & Thun, M.J. (2013). *Active smoking and breast cancer risk: original cohort data and meta-analysis. Journal of National Cancer Institute,105,515–525.*

Ghosh, R., Bank, S., Bhattacharya, R., Kahn, N.N. & Sinha, A.K. (2014). *Neutralization by Insulin of the Hypertensive Effect of Dermcidin Isoform 2: An Environmentally Induced Diabetogenic and Hypertensive Protein. Cardiology Research and Practice, Article ID 412815, doi.org/10.1155/2014/412815*

Ghosh, R., Bhattacharya, R., Bhattacharya, G. & Sinha, A.K. (2012). The Control of Stress Induced Type I Diabetes Mellitus in Humans through the Hepatic Synthesis of Insulin by the Stimulation of Nitric Oxide Production. International Journal of Biomedical Science, 8(3),171–182.

Ghosh, R., Jana, P. & Sinha, A.K. (2012). The Control of Hyperglycemia in Alloxan Treated Diabetic Mice through the Stimulation of Hepatic Insulin Synthesis due to the Production of Nitric Oxide. Experimental Clinical and Endocrinology Diabetes, 120(03),145–151.

Ghosh, R., Karmohapatra, S.K., Bhattacharya, G. & Sinha, A.K. (2010). The glucose-induced synthesis of insulin in liver. Endocrine, 38(2),294–302.

Ghosh, R., Karmohapatra, S.K., Bhattacharyya, M., Bhattacharya, R., Bhattacharya, G. & Sinha, A.K. (2011). The appearance of dermcidin isoform 2, a novel platelet aggregating agent in the circulation in acute myocardial infarction that inhibits insulin synthesis and the restoration by acetyl salicylic acid of its effects. Journal of Thrombosis and Thrombolysis, 31(1),13–21.

Ghosh, R., Maji, U.K., Bhattacharya, R., & Sinha, A.K. (2012). The Role of Dermcidin Isoform2: A Two-Faceted Atherosclerotic Risk Factor for Coronary Artery Disease and the Effect of Acetyl Salicylic Acid on It. Thrombosis, Article ID 987932 doi:10.1155/2012/987932.

Ghosh, R., Ray, U., Jana, P., Bhattacharya, R., Banerjee, D. & Sinha, A.K. (2014). Reduction of Death Rate Due to Acute Myocardial Infarction in Subjects with Cancers through Systemic Restoration of Impaired Nitric Oxide. PLoS ONE, 9(2),e88639.

Goldberg, I.J. (2001). Diabetic Dyslipidemia: Causes and Consequences. Journal of Clinical Endocrinology & Metabolism, 86(3),965–71.

Goldberg, R.J., Kramer, D.G., Lessard, D., Yarzebski, J. & Gore, J.M. (2007). Serum glucose levels and hospital outcomes in patients with acute myocardial infarction without prior diabetes: a community-wide perspective. Coronary Artery Disease, 18(2).125–131.

Hackett, P.H. & Roach, R.C. (2001). High-Altitude Illness. New England Journal of Medicine, 345,107–114.

Hughes, S.D., Johnson, J.H., Quaade, C. & Newgard, C.B. (1992). Engineering of glucose-stimulated insulin secretion and biosynthesis in non-islet cells. Proceedings of the National Academy of Sciences USA, 89(2),688–692.

Jia, L., Bonaventura, C., Bonaventura, J. & Stamler, J.S. (1996). S-nitrosohaemoglobin: a dynamic activity of blood involved in vascular control. Nature, 380,221–226.

Karmohapatra, S.K., Chakraborty, K., Kahn, N.N. & Sinha, A.K. (2003). Inhibition of human blood platelet aggregation and the stimulation of nitric oxide synthesis by aspirin. Platelets,14,421–427.

Karmohapatra, S.K., Chakraborty, K., Kahn, N.N. & Sinha, A.K. (2007). The role of nitric oxide in aspirin induced thrombolysis in vitro and the purification of aspirin activated nitric oxide synthase from human blood platelets. American Journal of Hematology, 82,986–995.

Klock, J.C. & Bainton, D.F. (1976). Degranulation and abnormal bactericidal function of *granulocytes procured by reversible adhesion to nylon wool. Blood, 48,149–161.*

Kojima, H., Fujimiya, M., Matsumura, K., Nakahara, T., Hara, M. & Chan, L. (2004). Extrapancreatic insulin producing cells in multiple organs in diabetes. Proceedings of the National Academy of Sciences USA, 101(8),2458–2463.

Kosiborod, M. (2008). Blood glucose and its prognostic implications in patients hospitalised with acute myocardial infarction. Diabetes and Vascular Disease Research, 5(4),269–275.

Libby, P. (2005). Prevention and treatment of atherosclerosis. In Harrison's Principles of Internal Medicine. pp.1430–1433.

Maritim, A.C., Sanders, R.A. & Watkins III, J.B. (2003). Diabetes, oxidative stress, and antioxidants: a review. Journal of Biochemical and Molecular Toxicology,17(1),24–38.

Maxwell, S.R.J. & Lip G.Y.H. (1997). Free radicals and antioxidants in cardiovascular disease. British Journal of Clinical Pharmacology, 44,307–317.

Page, D. L., Caulfield, J. B., Kastor, J. A., DeSanctis, R. W. & Sanders, C. A. (1971). Myocardial changes associated with cardiogenic shock. New England Journal of Medicine, 285, 133–7.

Pal, D., Dasgupta, S., Kundu, R., Maitra, S., Das, G., Mukhopadhyay, S., Ray, S., Majumdar, S.S. & Bhattacharya, S. (2012). Fetuin-A acts as an endogenous ligand of TLR4 to promote lipid-induced insulin resistance. Nature Medicine, 18(8),1279–85.Pfeifer, M.A., Halter, J.B. & Porte, D. (1981). Insulin secretion in diabetes mellitus. American Journal of Medicine, 70(3), 579–588.

Pollack, C.V. (1995). Emerging oral antiplatelet therapies for acute coronary syndromes. Hospital Practice, 38, 29–37.

Rathsman, B., Rosfors, S., Sjöholm, A. & Nyström, T. (2012). Early signs of atherosclerosis are associated with insulin resistance in non-obese adolescent and young adults with type 1 diabetes. Cardiovascular Diabetology, 27,11(145).

Sinha, A.K., Bhattacharya, S., Acharya, K. & Mazumder, S. (1999). Stimulation of nitric oxide synthesis and protective role of insulin in acute thrombosis in vivo. Life Science, 65,2687–2696.

Sowers, J.R., Epstein, M & Frohlich, E.D. (2001). Diabetes, hypertension, and cardiovascular disease an update. Hypertension, 37(4),1053–1059.

www.ingramcontent.com/pod-product-compliance
Lightning Source LLC
Chambersburg PA
CBHW081108220326
41598CB00038B/7279